"Alex Monk has written a monograph of great urgency and importance, both for the subtlety of its argumentation and its sensitivity to neglected aspects of psychic life. Modernity can no longer pretend that magical consciousness is an artifact of the past, and Monk's work triumphs in recommending the integration, rather than the denial, of the weirdness that will not go away."

—**J. F. Martel,** author of *Reclaiming Art in the Age of Artifice* and co-host of the *Weird Studies* Podcast

"The curse is a powerful image evoking the inexorable workings of an unseen force that works against us, thwarts our efforts, and condemns us to suffering and struggle. It's a fascinating lens through which to explore clinical work with those individuals who seem perpetually dogged by the dark forces in their own unconscious. This volume artfully ties the age-old, archetypal language of the curse to psychoanalytic thought, providing a unique perspective that brings additional insights to familiar clinical issues."

—**Lisa Marchiano,** Jungian analyst and author of *Motherhood: Facing and Finding Yourself*

"Alex Monk's comparative approach is a much welcome development in psychoanalysis. His psychoanalytic perspective on the 'evil eye' phenomenon illustrates the importance of locating clinical work within cross-cultural contexts that also attend to multiple social factors such as economics and class. Monk's clinical presentations are especially compelling as he reflects upon the impact his patients have on him."

—**Marsha Aileen Hewitt,** University of Toronto, author of *Freud on Religion* and *Legacies of the Occult: Psychoanalysis, Religion, and Unconscious Communication*

Trauma and the Supernatural in Psychotherapy

Trauma and the Supernatural in Psychotherapy explores how traumatic experience interacts with unconscious phantasy based in folklore, the supernatural, and the occult.

Drawing upon psychoanalysis, anthropology, the arts, and esoteric philosophy, Alex Monk presents examples from folklore and literature to enrich his case illustrations which offer therapists important clinical perspectives on ways of working with clients who feel cursed and repeatedly manifest self-sabotaging states. The book examines the challenges that can arise when working with this client population and illustrates how to work through them while navigating potent transferences and projective identifications. Monk illustrates the way in which clients with developmental trauma may experience the supernatural and its psychic representatives as persecutory and/or a source of empowerment and healing. *Trauma and the Supernatural in Psychotherapy* also considers the historically conflicted relationship between psychoanalysis and the supernatural and proposes treatment perspectives which are not implicitly dependent upon a materialist paradigm.

This book will be of great interest to psychotherapists and counsellors who have an interest in clinical work concerning the connection of relational trauma to unconscious forms of communication and uncanny phenomena arising between therapist and client.

Alex Monk is an integrative arts psychotherapist and musician based in London, UK. He has a private practice in East London. He has a particular interest in psychoanalysis; the arts; and the weird, uncanny, and magical.

Trauma and the Supernatural in Psychotherapy

Working with the Curse Position in Clinical Practice

Alex Monk

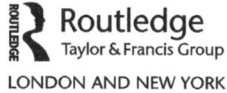

Routledge
Taylor & Francis Group

LONDON AND NEW YORK

Designed cover image: Newark Cemetery by Jennifer Holt.
Instagram @jennypenwren

First published 2023
by Routledge
4 Park Square, Milton Park, Abingdon, Oxon OX14 4RN

and by Routledge
605 Third Avenue, New York, NY 10158

*Routledge is an imprint of the Taylor & Francis Group, an informa
business*

© 2023 Alex Monk

British Library Cataloguing-in-Publication Data
A catalogue record for this book is available from the British Library

ISBN: 978-0-367-76672-6 (hbk)
ISBN: 978-0-367-70747-7 (pbk)
ISBN: 978-1-003-16802-7 (ebk)

DOI: 10.4324/9781003168027

Typeset in Times New Roman
by Apex CoVantage, LLC

For Serenella.

Contents

Acknowledgements

Thank you first and foremost to my clients who have taught me so much. Thank you to my wife and family for all their encouragement and patience throughout this process. I would like to thank the late Chris Mawson for his generous and gracious suggestions and for encouraging me to write this book. Thanks to the UKCP Practitioner Research Network for feedback on my ideas. I am extremely grateful to my readers Alistair Stevenson, Natalie Kennedy, Carl Taylor, and Kate Hardwicke for offering their time and insightful comments. Thank you also to all the team at Routledge, the *Weird Studies* podcast for your inspirational conversations, J.F. Martel, Lisa Marchiano, Marsha Hewitt, Vanessa Sinclair, Will Kearney, Barry Watt, Geraldine Monk, Mark Stone, and Andrew Rowe.

Introduction

The Foundations of the Curse Position Theory

I observed a pattern in my clinical work where clients felt themselves to be the victim of a disproportionate amount of bad luck yet could never account for why this was the case. They were usually aware that this self-perception had become a self-fulfilling prophecy but felt powerless to break its spell. Aside from this misfortune of inexplicable origin, I also came across cases where the bad luck would be attributed to the *maleficent* intent of another individual. The client would thus perceive that being friends with, or merely associating with this particular person was in itself a cause of misfortune – though once again, could not usually offer a 'rational' explanation for it. Nevertheless, aside from occasional exceptions, the client did not 'really' feel that they were 'cursed' with bad luck or that the person with malicious intent 'actually' had supernatural powers, yet what they were telling me was clearly important, and it troubled them.

After working through various hypotheses, I began to wonder whether what my clients described indicated an 'unthought known', somehow of *supernatural* origin (Bollas, 2018). As the clients who felt this way had also often experienced relational trauma, I therefore hypothesised that the affective experience which they struggled to communicate was somehow the result of a strange alchemy between developmental trauma and this 'supernatural' internal object that could not be thought about. I was also struck by the way that the very particular feeling they described felt so familiar – a sense of being 'at home' – yet was equally experienced as a returning impingement on subjectivity and – perhaps most importantly – always threatened to do so.

I didn't know it at the time, but I would later realise that what my clients were describing was a discordant convergence of the *heimlich* and the *unheimlich*, the homely and the unhomely – otherwise known as Freud's 'uncanny' (1919). Yet I did not make this vital connection with Freud's seminal essay until after I had read Mark Fisher's *Ghosts of My Life*. I was quickly awestruck by the way in which Fisher seemed to uniquely apprehend the phenomenon that my clients described, noting that whether one believes 'in the supernatural or not, the family is a haunted structure' (Fisher, 2014, p. 43). It was clear that Fisher understood the essence of haunted and cursed subjectivity.

DOI: 10.4324/9781003168027-1

In *The Uncanny*, Freud describes a *daimonic* compulsion to repeat (1919). Initially it appears that Freud's *daimon* is a sabotaging entity of supernatural origin, yet, as his essay is framed in a materialist paradigm, he therefore dismisses the archaic unconscious as essentially 'primitive', thereby closing the door on its mysterious and nuanced vistas (Freud, 1919). I therefore felt it was important to seek out historical and anthropological perspectives on this relationship between misfortune and the supernatural and, in doing so, came across Ronald Hutton's *The Witch*. Hutton's monograph proved instructive as he points to a universal, archaic fear of attack by supernatural means or 'uncanny misfortune' (2017). This therefore helps to account for the 'unthought known' that I have described, driven by an arcane fear in the depths of one's unconscious that the cause of one's misfortune is a supernatural bad object: a curse. Hutton also points to a common historical tendency to attribute the cause of this 'uncanny misfortune' to others, which provides us with important data for the projective phenomenon I have described (ibid.). I therefore began to consider that if it is indeed the case that there is a universal fear of uncanny attack, this may well be significantly amplified with clients who have experienced developmental trauma, given that they already inhabit a universe in which threat is experienced as an emergency (Van der Kolk, 1989). These combined elements came to form the basis of the theory of 'the curse position'.

After developing the core theory of the curse position, I then began to look at further perspectives on the way in which trauma relates to the supernatural. As Donald Kalsched elucidates in *The Inner World of Trauma* – which has also been an important influence on my clinical thinking – traumatised individuals often exhibit a unique sensitivity and mythopoetic imagination yet are also troubled by destructive unconscious phantasies and cruel superegos which relate to the depth of their attachment wounds (Kalsched, 1996). The 'mythopoetic' imagination that Kalsched points to therefore provides a theoretical basis for the supernatural currents which drive the unconscious phantasies of the curse position. This imaginative capacity is part of what I refer to in this book as 'magical consciousness', and I propose that it may have its origins in what Ferenczi calls the traumatised infant's 'clairvoyant' relationship to the caregiver (Ferenczi, 1988). This 'clairvoyance' may become a source of psychopathology or be harnessed for creativity and psycho-spiritual growth, each of which can be symbolised by the two aspects of the *daimon* as posited by Jung (1979).

A Note on Terminology and Case Vignettes

I use the word 'position' rather than 'syndrome' to emphasise the psychological and affective 'place' to which the individual periodically returns. I wish to emphasise, however, that the curse position is not intended as a diagnostic term.

Aside from the case illustrations, with the objective of maintaining consistency of style, I refer to clients as 'she', to the therapist as 'he', and to the child as 'she' unless otherwise stated. I have used case vignettes to illustrate relevant clinical theory, and in the interest of protecting confidentiality, I have presented examples which consist of composite clients. As the accompanying therapeutic interventions, dialogues, and countertransference analyses relate to these composite cases, they are therefore essentially works of fiction, yet my intention is that they nonetheless illustrate the pertinent presenting issues and themes that arise in the consulting room and my clinical approach to them. The dreams that I have presented in the case illustrations are also fictional examples, though they are intended to convey the atmospheric and thematic qualities of dreams that clients have reported to me over the years. My encounter with the uncanny during the coronavirus pandemic (detailed in chapter 4) and the memory I have used as an example of reverie (chapter 10) are both events I personally experienced.

References

Bollas, C. (2018). *The Shadow of the Object. Psychoanalysis of the Unthought Known*. London: Routledge.

Ferenczi, S. (1988). Confusion of tongues between adults and the child – The language of tenderness and of passion. *Contemporary Psychoanalysis*, 24: 196–206.

Fisher, M. (2014). *Ghosts of My Life: Writings on Depression, Hauntology and Lost Futures*. Winchester: Zero Books.

Freud, S. (1919). The 'Uncanny'. In Freud, A., Strachey, A., Strachey, J, and Tyson A. (Eds.), *The Standard Edition of the Complete Psychological Works of Sigmund Freud, Volume XVII (1917–1919): An Infantile Neurosis and Other Works*. London: Hogarth Press, pp. 217–256.

Hutton, R. (2017). *The Witch*. New Haven: Yale University Press.

Jung, C. G. L. (1979). *Aion: Researches into the Phenomenology of the Self*. Princeton: Princeton University Press.

Kalsched, D. (1996). *The Inner World of Trauma: Archetypal Defenses of the Personal Spirit*. London: Routledge.

Van der Kolk, B. A. (1989). The compulsion to repeat the trauma: Re-enactment, revictimization, and masochism. *Psychiatric Clinics of North America*, 12(2): 389–411.

Chapter 1

Magic and the Supernatural

The Historical Context
for the Curse Position

Introduction

The aim of this chapter acts as a context setting for the chapters to follow and provides the foundation for the subsequent chapters that focus on the clinical and theoretical material to which it relates.

> Attributing the uncanny nature of misfortune to random chance alone is often insufficient: people generally wish to attribute bad luck to the 'human or super-human' agencies.
>
> (Hutton, 2017, p. 10)

As Hutton suggests, there is an important human relationship among the super-natural, fate, and (mis)fortune. Given the fear and sense of powerlessness associated with the possibility of becoming harmed through supernatural means, over time individuals have resorted to magical and cursing practises as a source of regaining that power and seeking revenge.

Along with the fear of supernatural entities, there has been a concomitant anxiety around those who are believed to use magic for uncanny means, such as the Persian *magi* and the 'witches' of medieval and early modern Europe. As will become clear throughout this chapter, magic and the supernatural have been successively othered, in the name of either religion or scientific progress, for millennia. Moreover, in psychoanalysis and psychotherapy, numinous, intuitive, and uncanny states of mind have become all too easily be conflated with 'magical thinking' and associated with psychopathology, 'primitive' cultures, and omnipotent thought. These divisive factors have contributed to a collectively split mind where magic and supernatural experiences are either idealised or experienced as persecutory. I therefore propose that numinous, uncanny, and intuitive phenomenology fall under the term 'magical consciousness'.

This chapter also explores movements throughout history which have sought to reintegrate this magical consciousness into its societies such as the Renaissance, the 'Magical Revival' of the *fin de siècle*, and contemporary 'occulture' (Partridge, 2004–2005). Despite the unavoidably complicated relationship between magic and

DOI: 10.4324/9781003168027-2

trauma – an important theme for this book – these examples of synthesis also become significant factors in terms of potentially healing the splits that have formed in the archaic unconscious.

The Ancient Context: Uncanny Misfortune

There is very little doubt that in every inhabited continent of the world, the majority of recorded human societies have believed in, and feared, an ability by some individuals to cause misfortune and injury to others by nonphysical and uncanny ('magical') means.
—Hutton, 2017, p. 10

Here, Hutton indicates the universality of a fear of intended harm by magical means. Indeed, the potency of this fear is not to be underestimated: Walter Cannon (1942) demonstrates, through his research across a range of geographical and cross-cultural settings, the way in which the fight-or-flight response can be triggered. His anthropological studies show that fear of an uncanny attack or the perceived breaking of a social taboo may lead to the actual 'voodoo' death of the subject (ibid.).

Bever's later research also notes the link between the fear and aggression of supernatural attack and the neurobiological harm it may cause (2008, p. 25). As hostility is transmitted not only verbally but also through gaze and prosody, this also has significant implications for the extent to which hostile affects are introjected unknowingly (ibid.).[1] This therefore has an important bearing on projective identification and countertransference, both of which are often reported by psychotherapists to be transmitted unconsciously.[2]

I now provide examples of cultural factors in the ancient world which could have contributed to this fear which now resides in an archaic unconscious, populated by disturbing entities which overwhelm the subject, particularly in cases of trauma. This archaic unconscious provides the foundational level of the curse position.

Mesopotamia

The spirituality of Mediterranean culture in the ancient world was replete with supernatural entities, and its population consisted of a wide range of demons, gods, angels, and ghosts to contend with (Gager, 1992, p. 12). This abundance of deities and supernatural phenomena particularly applied to Ancient Mesopotamia (modern-day Iraq). As a result of the use of cuneiform (script imprinted on clay tablets), many magical texts survive from this period (Geller, 1997; Maxwell-Stuart, 2017).

Mesopotamians attributed significant powers to gods and demonic entities which were myriad and held responsible for the onset of disease and misfortune (Hutton, 2017, p. 48). Adverse events in one's life were therefore either caused by offending an angry god or by the malicious intent of a demon (Geller, 1997). An awareness of fate and its omens was a part of everyday life in Mesopotamian society, and it is this aspect which is of particular relevance to the curse position, as I have found this preoccupation to also be common in clients who have suffered from relational trauma. As will become clear in Chapter 3, there is therefore an important interplay between the archaic unconscious, unconscious phantasy, and relational trauma.

Another important aspect of the curse position which recurs throughout this book is that of a malign, or *demonic*, superego. The following description of the widely feared Sumerian (Mesopotamian) demons known as the *Maskim* evokes the qualities of this kind of out-of-control conscience: *Maskim* is a literal translation of 'bailiff': 'the demonic equivalent to a corrupt official, against whom one is virtually powerless' (Geller, 1997, p. 2). When one considers the particular savagery of the superego that results from relational trauma, the inherent powerlessness the Mesopotamian citizen experienced when confronted by this demonic bailiff becomes allegorically pertinent.

Given the menacing nature of the supernatural world in Mesopotamia, the use of divinatory and sympathetic magic became an important means of defending against the caprice of demons and gods. This important magical praxis was conducted by a designated priest called the *ašipu* (Hutton, 2017, p. 48; Seligman, 2018, p. 24). With the adoption of the religion of Zoroaster, the Mesopotamian pantheon was divided into two entities: the 'good' creator Ormazd and the 'evil' Ahriman who were in mutual conflict. All other deities were therefore subsumed into a hierarchical system as either angels or demons of their assigned entity (Hutton, 2017, p. 50; Seligman, 2018, p. 40). Insects and flies were then classified as demonic agents of Ahriman, as they were believed to be born of corruption (rather than semen) as 'nothing imperfect could derive from Ormazd' (Seligman, 2018, p. 44). This Zoroastrian demonisation of flies is the genesis of *The Lord of the Flies* or *Beelzebub* found in Judaism and Christianity (Seligman, 2018, p. 47). This dualistic development therefore becomes an important contributory factor in compounding the split in the archaic unconscious and the resultant malevolence of its demons and holier-than-thou nature of its angels.

Egypt

For the Ancient Egyptians, religion and magic were one and the same, and this also applied to priest and magician (Hutton, 2017, p. 46). The boundary between Egyptian civilisation and its deities was 'porous', and they were unified by *heka* (the Egyptian word for magic), 'signifying the animating and controlling force of the universe' (Hutton, 2017, p. 45). *Heka* is a 'magical vitality' which permeates creation, and with its power comes the capacity to curse, exorcise, and protect (Maxwell-Stuart, 2017, p. 6). Importantly, *heka* binds magic to the spoken and the written word (ibid.). Indeed, for the Ancient Egyptians, all words had a magical effect, not only those uttered in incantations (Seligman, 2018, p. 69). The way in which individuals were named in Ancient Egypt betrays this magical essence of the word as a symbol: babies were assigned two names at birth: a 'lesser' name, which was publicly known, and the 'greater name' – that of the *ka* (spirit-double) – which was kept secret and 'embodied all the individual's magical power' (Seligman, 2018, p. 68).

Israel-Judaea-Palestine

As Maxwell-Stuart (2017, p. 12) writes, 'Israel-Judaea-Palestine was open to [magical] influences from Mesopotamia and Egypt, which included not only the kinds of operation we have seen already in its neighbours', but according to Seligman, 'divination of future and hidden things gained the strongest foothold in Israel' (2018, p. 55).

There are two well-known examples of divinatory magic in the Old Testament, and in their own way, each features a supernatural entity that holds the keys to a human being's fate.

Firstly, in the story of the Witch of Endor (1 Samuel 28:9; King James Version), King Saul consults a familiar (helping) spirit after Yahweh's refusal to advise him. The spirit (the prophet Samuel) then 'confronted the terrified king with his approaching death' (ibid.). As Seligman points out, it is subject to exegesis whether the familiar spirit was an agent of God sent to scare Saul or a 'phantom from hell' (ibid.).

The second example is that of the 'scapegoat' found in Leviticus 16:8–10. On the Day of Atonement, the high priest Aaron cast lots over two goats: one is offered to Yahweh for sacrifice, 'but the scapegoat that was Azazel's, they sent into the wilderness with the sins of Israel' (Seligman, 2018, p. 55). Azazel is a demonic entity, and this ceremony therefore connects the sins of the populace (guilt) with evil.[3] Jungian analyst Sylvia Perera notes the archetypal nature of the scapegoat ceremony and the concomitant role of guilt, a *shameful evil*. This understandably contributes to an intractable 'scapegoat complex':

> individuals identified with the scapegoat archetype feel themselves to be the carriers of shamefully evil behaviours and attitudes that disrupt relationships.
>
> (Perera, 1986, p. 15)

Ancient Greece

The word 'magic' originates from the Greek *mageia*, derived from the Persian *magos*, which refers to the rituals and practices of the Chaldean (now Persian) 'fire' priests/magicians in the fifth century BCE (Davies, 2012, p. 1, Maxwell-Stuart, 2017, p. 18). However, as these elite priests did not themselves practice magic, the dim view that the Greeks[4] held towards magical practice was instead driven by a distrust of 'foreigners', fuelled by memories of Zoroastrian occupation (Maxwell-Stuart, 2017, p. 18). Magic was therefore considered by the Greek establishment to be a nefarious pursuit only practised by 'alien sorcerers' (Ogden, 2002), despite its widespread use (Maxwell-Stuart, 2017, p. 20). These double standards are underscored by Homer's *Odyssey*, which is full of magical operations and which would have been completed 'long before the Greeks had even heard of the Persians' (Ogden, 2002, p. 33).

Aside from *mageia*, the Greeks also practised *goetia* – sorcery – and *pharmakeia*, a curative medicinal magic which utilised herbs and potions of both a curative and poisonous nature (Maxwell-Stuart, 2017, pp. 18–19). A well-known example of the magical control of *goetic* demons is found in the 17th century *grimoire The Lesser Key of Solomon*, where King Solomon is reported to harness the power of 72 demons through the use of a magic ring (Mistlberger, 2020, p. 255). The more benign *daimonian* is also born in Ancient Greece, a Platonic familiar spirit which mediates between the natural and divine worlds (Plutarch et al., 2010). Although *daimones* would typically 'speak' to individuals in dreams, a gifted individual such as Socrates was able to apprehend his guiding spirit even when awake (Russell, 2010, p. 3). The *daimonian* is therefore also concerned with intuition and fate.

Ancient Rome

Historical records from Mesopotamia, Israel-Judaea-Palestine, Egypt, and Greece show that magic was principally conducted by men, yet in Ancient Rome, the female magician becomes much more prevalent in poetry and satirical literature (Maxwell-Stuart, 2017, p. 25). Greek witches, such as Homer's 'fair tressed' Circe, are generally described as 'young and beautiful', yet their Roman counterparts, such as Horace's Canidia, are 'old and ugly' (Stanley Spaeth, 2014, p. 46). The 'evil' of magic was therefore now not only projected into other cultures but also women. Thus, it is in Ancient Rome where we can locate the early indicators of scapegoating women as 'evil' and held responsible for uncanny misfortune: fear is defended against by aggression.

Binding Curses

When the Egyptian civilisation became part of the Roman empire, there was a continued distrust of magic and its practitioners along with the dissociation of religion from magic, signified by the latter civilisation's passing of draconian laws against it (Hutton, 2017, p. 102). By the second century CE, magic had become associated with *maleficium*: the deliberate cause of harm to other citizens (Hutton, 2017, p. 61). With the consequent closure of Egyptian temples and the limited scope of its priests to practice magic, there was also a need to adapt in order to continue the dissemination of knowledge and ritual– hence, the emergence of the 'magical papyri', texts which contained 'recipes' for a form of sympathetic magic known as a 'binding curse' which would ' "bind" or "restrain" an intended victim' (Hutton, 2017, p. 102; Ogden, 2002, p. 210).

Despite the Roman disdain for magical practice, 'binding curses' (*defixiones* in Latin) were widespread in the empire, spanning from Egypt to Britain (Ogden, 2002, p.7). As John Gager writes, 'Everyone, it seems, used or knew of them' (1992, p. 3). The curses were commonly etched onto small pieces of iron or lead which were sometimes folded and nailed down in a sympathetic representation of the restraint of the intended victim (Ogden, 2002, p. 210). The tablets would utilise *voces magicae* and palindromes in order to increase their magical potency and appeal to the demon that would carry out the curse (Gager, 1992; Ogden, 2002). Curse tablets were buried underground or in a location close to the targeted recipient (Ogden, 2002). 'Voodoo dolls' were an earlier, less common, image-based version of the binding curse. Small 'poppets' were created to represent the victim, and their limbs were bound or their bodies twisted into symbolically agonising positions, hammered down onto a hard surface with nails, or placed inside tiny coffins. Sometimes the name of the spell intended for the victim was also inscribed on the doll itself (Ogden, 2002, p. 245).

Magic & Religion

Christians were among those at risk of persecution in the second century Roman Empire for invoking sprits by magical means, known as 'ceremonial magic' (Hutton, 2017, p. 148). Since miracles attributed to Jesus could easily be construed as 'magical', this meant that Christ's followers were vulnerable to pagan accusations of the same (ibid.). This, in turn, led to Christians needing to find their own means of establishing a separate identity by using the same splitting strategy to those in the Graeco-Roman empire. In the third century, Christian theologians such as Origen therefore unfavourably compared the rites and incantations of ceremonial magicians with those of 'authentic' Christians, who employed only the words of the bible and the name of Jesus (Hutton, 2017, p. 148).

The increased interest in ceremonial magic in the 12th century was also generated by an awareness that Islamic and Jewish cultures had retained philosophical links with privileged knowledge from the world of antiquity that Christianity had lost (Davies, 2012, p. 42). A notable example of this was the Arabic *grimoire Ġhāyat al-Ḥakīm – The Aim of the Sage* – translated into Latin as *The Picatrix* (Gager, 1992; Page, 2017; Williams, 2020). The magician Caraphzebiz is described in *The Picatrix* as the 'founder of magic' and the first magus to have a familiar spirit who

> performed marvels for him, helped him understand the secrets of nature and the sciences, and came when invoked with sacrifices.
>
> (Page, 2017, p. 36)

As a result of the discovery of *The Picatrix* and the increased use of ceremonial magic among Christians in the medieval and early modern periods, there was now a resurgent need for magicians who could use demons for divine ends in order to favourably differentiate themselves from 'witches', whose work was seen the result of a pact with Satan (Hutton, 2017, p. 99; Williams, 2020, p. 97). As a result of these actions, this meant that non-Christian faiths were also vulnerable to accusations of witchcraft: Jews, for example, needed to 'rein in' certain customs for fear of persecution, as Jewish ceremonial magic was not considered acceptable to the Christian church (Trachtenberg, 2013).

Witchcraft

The contributory historical factors which have combined to inculcate a collective dread of uncanny misfortune and *maleficium* are complex and nuanced, yet some possible sources of this have by now become clear. The Mesopotamian dread of demons and subsequent Zoroastrian split between good and evil became important antecedents of the Judeo-Christian dualism that was to follow. In the Graeco-Roman world, magic was considered a nefarious pursuit practised by 'alien sorcerers' such as Babylonians, Egyptians, and – in Ancient Rome – women. With the publication of the theologian St. Augustine of Hippo's *City of God* in the fifth century CE, all spiritual beliefs outside of Christianity had become tantamount to witchcraft (Callow, 2018 p. 56). This text became a significant source of inspiration for Heinrich Kramer's highly influential 15th century text *Malleus Maleficarum* (*The Hammer of Witches*), which, in turn, was used by 'witchfinders' to persecute those practising *maleficium* (ibid.). By now, the Christian notion of the pact between the Devil and the witch as his servant had become widespread, and the propaganda of *Malleus Maleficarum* entrenched fear and loathing among the public, contributing to the death of between 40,000 and 60,000 people across Europe between 1560 and 1640, many of whom were women (Hutton, 2017 p. 180; Williams, 2020, p. 97). Nevertheless, the attribution of *maleficium* to witches or their cultural equivalents is a global phenomenon, and witches have been associated with 'incest, nudity and cannibalism' in areas as diverse as Nigeria, Polynesia, Indonesia, and Thailand (Hutton, 2017, pp. 22–23).

All of these examples point to the disavowal of a chthonic, shadow self which has been defended against by projecting it into other groups or individuals who are often powerless to defend themselves. This unconscious threat is linked to the sense of disproportionate injustice and victimisation that are important aspects of the phenomenology of the curse position illustrated in subsequent chapters. These examples also point to the link between fear and aggression, where fear of one's own destructive urges is projected into the other as *maleficium*, resulting in one's disavowed aggression nonetheless acted out in unjust acts of persecution and scapegoating.

Neoplatonism and the Renaissance

In his highly influential text *Religion and the Decline of Magic*, Keith Thomas pinpoints Neoplatonism's popularity as a determining factor of establishing a magical 'reboot' in the Western world. Neoplatonism advocated the sympathetic fusion of matter and spirit – *as above, so below*. According to Thomas, there was now a burgeoning belief that all elements of the universe contained magical properties and that the world of spirits could be accessed once again (1971, p. 265). The Neoplatonists found an associated sympathy between Pythagorean geometry and divinatory practices such as astrology and palmistry, also benefitting from a climate where the imagination could uncover the occult secrets of the spirit world (Thomas,

1971, p. 266). This therefore heralded a return to the merging of the material and supernatural worlds that had taken place in Ancient Egypt. The Renaissance also saw the publication of Ficino's Latin translation of the *Corpus Hermeticum*, which was believed to have predated Christianity and Plato and contained teachings from the Ancient Egyptian god Hermes Trismegistus (Thomas, 1971, p. 267).

> Its astrological and alchemical lore helped to create an intellectual environment sympathetic to every kind of mystical and magical activity.
>
> (Thomas, 1971, p. 267)

The Renaissance therefore synthesised natural and spiritual phenomena, once again accompanied by an eagerness to embrace a range of disciplines and philosophies, one of which would have a significant importance for Jung: alchemy. Jung describes the way in which the alchemical *coniunctio* offers a means of overcoming the duality of monotheistic religion:

> rather like an undercurrent to the Christianity that ruled on the surface. It is to this surface that the dream is to consciousness, and just as the dream contemplates the conscious mind, so alchemy endeavours to fill in the gaps left open by the Christian tension of opposites.
>
> (Jung, 1968, p. 23)

According to Thomas, however, by the late 17th century, the starry-eyed union of science and magic that the Renaissance had kickstarted was now in sharp decline (p. 770).

> Magnetism and electricity, which had previously been seen as occult influences, could now be explained in purely mechanical terms as the movement of particles. The triumph of the mechanical philosophy meant the end of the animistic conception of the universe which had constituted the basic rationale for magical thinking.
>
> (Thomas, 1971, p. 771)

Thomas paints a world which parallels the disenchantment thesis of the German anthropologist Max Weber:

> The fate of our times is characterized by rationalization and intellectualization and, above all, by the 'disenchantment of the world'.
>
> (Weber, in Josephson-Storm, 2017, p. 269)

Josephson-Storm refutes the thesis of Thomas and Weber: for Josephson-Storm, magic never went away, and some of the key 'scapegoats' of disenchantment (Bacon, Bruno, Newton, et al.) 'saw themselves as magicians' (Josephson-Storm, 2017, p. 41). Despite these important caveats, the 1890 publication of J.G. Frazer's

The Golden Bough introduced a new anthropological imperialism which drew a neat, though arbitrary, line of progress between magical, religious, and scientific civilisations. *The Golden Bough* was also an influential text for Freud, particularly with regard to his writing on the 'omnipotence of thoughts', which would become widely referred to psychoanalytically as 'magical thinking' (Freud, 1960). Freud locates magical thinking in the pre-Oedipal stage of development and regards it as a regressive tendency in adults which manifests in paranoia and obsessional neurosis (ibid.). Freud thus presents an analogue in the human developmental stages to Frazer's anthropological thesis, moving from the 'omnipotence of thoughts' (narcissism) through to religion (object choice) and finally to the pinnacle of scientific endeavour and renunciation of the pleasure principle (Freud, 1960, p. 90).

It is my view that regressive and omnipotent defences present themselves frequently clinically, particularly in cases of relational trauma, and the term 'magical thinking' (when 'psychic reality eclipses external reality') is therefore apposite to describe a psychic process where unconscious phantasy hijacks the external world, and, as we will see, this is prevalent as a defence in the curse position (Ogden, 2010, p. 321). However, the association of the term with the evolutionary/developmental paradigm of Frazer and Freud is ethically problematic, as this perspective relegates 'primitive' ontological experience to an inferior category (Frazer and Fraser, 1994; Freud, 1960). Furthermore, experiences of the uncanny, synchronicity, nostalgia, and precognition can all too easily be subsumed into the category of magical thinking. I would therefore propose the use of the alternative term 'magical consciousness' to describe experiences of the former. Greenwood and Goodwyn define magical consciousness as follows:

> A relational and holistic aspect of the mind in which spiritual entities are experienced as pervading the universe, magical consciousness, as we are using the term, differs from logical, abstract, and analytical thinking, the more usual focus of cognitive science.
>
> (2016, p. xvi)

Along with the perhaps more obvious experiences one would associate with magical consciousness, such as synchronicity and the uncanny, Greenwood and Goodwyn importantly also highlight the *affective* aspect of magical consciousness and what is phenomenologically experienced as *subjectively meaningful*. For Jung, this 'affectivity' is 'the central organising principle of psychic life' (Kalsched, 1996, p. 88). Affect is also central to Bion's psychoanalytic paradigm, from which Ogden develops his concept of 'transformative thinking':

> In transformative thinking, one creates new ways of ordering experience in which not only new meanings, but new types of feeling, forms of object relatedness, and qualities of emotional and bodily aliveness are generated.
>
> (Ogden, 2010, p. 230)

An additional aspect of magical consciousness is its fostering of a profound connection to intuition, as here defined by Bergson scholar Wildon Carr:

> That sympathetic attitude to the reality without us that makes us seem to enter into it, to be with it, to live with it.
>
> (Wildon Carr, 2004, p. 45)

As relational trauma leaves the individual alienated and often in conflict with affective and intuitive aspects of ontology, magical consciousness offers a potential source of a renewed connection with them as additional resources to one's existing thinking apparatus, fostering greater harmony between thoughts and feelings as well as endogenous and veridical reality. It is important to note – in order not to promote a splitting or dualistic approach – that clients may bring psychic experiences into the consulting room which contain elements of *both* magical thinking and consciousness. These are not always easy to tell apart, and it is therefore tempting to fall into a trap of pathologising one or idealising the other.

The Magical Revival

As we have seen, Freud locates a 'primitive' magical mind in the archaic unconscious and posits that we experience its residue in uncanny experiences[5] (Freud, 1919). One may well therefore speculate that the archaic unconscious posed both a fascination and a threat to him, and, as we will see from the following chapter, he would carry this ambivalence with him for much of his life. Could the neat evolution Freud therefore posits in *Totem and Taboo* have been his own means of defence against the uncanny threat of the supernatural, where he substitutes scientific 'progress' for religious dogma? Aleister Crowley – a counterculture figure who embodied the aforementioned fusion of magical thinking and consciousness – is scathing in this regard:

> It is evident that the errors of the Unconscious of which the psycho-analysts complain are neither more nor less than the 'original sin' of the theologians whom they despise so heartily.
>
> (Crowley, 1991, p. xxiv)

Josephson-Storm (2017) notes that Crowley cites a section of *The Golden Bough* – the same text Freud uses to posit his evolutionary/developmental theory – to emphasise the parity between magic and science.

> Thus the analogy between the magical and the scientific conceptions of the world is close. In both of them the succession of events is perfectly regular and certain.
>
> (Frazer in Crowley, 1991, p. x)

Although Aleister Crowley loathed monotheistic religion, he saw magic and science as complementary disciplines. Crowley and the fellow occultists of the early 20th century may have shared Freud's view that the magical unconscious is antecedent to an evolutionary system. However, rather than reducing it to a more 'primitive' form of consciousness, its knowledge, rituals, and entities are considered sacred and deeply revered.

The magical practice of Ancient Egypt was a key reference point for Western occultists and to Crowley's 'New Gnosis of Light' of *Thelema* (the law of true will), which was dictated to him by 'a praeter-human Intelligence named Aiwaz' on his visit to Cairo in 1904 (Grant, 1972, p. 7).

Crowley's former secretary and fellow occultist Kenneth Grant shared Crowley's belief that the end of the 19th century heralded an era where the 'strands [of science and occultism] were gathered together and tied in a single knot' (Grant, 1972, p. 8). Grant pinpoints 1875 as the year when two events 'of far reaching importance' coincided: the birth of Crowley and the foundation of the Theosophical Society (ibid.). The Theosophical Society was formed by Madame Blavatsky and her associate Colonel Henry Steel Olcott, and it drew upon Western philosophy and Eastern mysticism (Owen, 2004, p. 29). Like Crowley, Blavatsky used her skills as a medium to channel ancient and esoteric knowledge, though her sources were of Indian rather than Egyptian origin, known to her as the 'Mahatmas' – the Masters (Owen, 2004, p. 310). Theosophy would also be an influence on artists such as Hilma af Klimt and Georgiana Houghton, who would channel spirits as a core aspect of their creative process.

Other societies of note that contributed to the magical revival were The Hermetic Order of the Golden Dawn and Crowley's incarnation of the Ordo Templi Orientis. Grant emphasises the anti-Christian current of Western esotericism in the magical revival (1972, p. 8). Importantly, Francis King points out that

> their foundation came at a time when many people were beginning to become dissatisfied with the pathetically over-confident materialism of the nineteenth century science on one hand, and the fatuous pietism of fundamentalist religion on the other.
>
> (1989, p. 44)

The adepts of these societies used ceremonial magic as a means of communicating with spirits, though it would be a highly gifted artist and magician who would revolutionise this approach.

Austin Osman Spare: an Atavistic Resurgence

Austin Osman Spare, a former member of Crowley's Argenteum Astrum (Order of the Silver Star), created a simple and innovative form of 'sigil magic'. Unlike ceremonial magic, Spare's method requires little paraphernalia and harnesses the power of the unconscious to do the magician's bidding. The magical practitioner clearly sets an intention and then creates a *sigil* (a magical symbol) which represents the desired outcome; then, most importantly, in order for it to be effective, the magician must forget his/her wish. Spare held that the hieroglyphs of Ancient Egypt and the Native Americans are 'the remainder of an occult knowledge' (Grant, 2011, p. xxvi) which can be accessed through an 'atavistic resurgence' (Baker, 2011, p. 90). The ritual 'charging' of the sigil or the use of automatic writing enables the practitioner to bypass the 'censor' of the ego and access the unconscious or, as Spare poetically calls it, 'the storehouse of memories with an ever-open door' (Spare, 2011, p. 47). Clearly, for Spare, like Jung, the archaic unconscious becomes a means of transcending duality. This results in Spare's *Kia*, 'expressed in words as the Neither-Neither' (Spare, 2011, p. 7), which one may compare to the *atman* and the Tao (Baker, 2011).

Concluding Comments

For Spare, like Jung, magical consciousness and its familiar spirits are to be embraced. However, as we have seen from the historical examples of this chapter, perhaps as a result of a universal fear of magic and the supernatural and their association with the deepest and most chaotic layers of the mind, they have presented a particular threat to those in power and have therefore been split off and defended against in various ways.

The magical revival proved to be a significant cultural movement which forged a new *fin de siècle* occult tradition which is explored in the next chapter in the light of concurrent advances in psychology, science, and technology. The occult movement of the *fin de siècle* has also been a considerable influence on related spiritual practices leading to the contemporary era, where a neo-magical renaissance is in full swing, with movements such as Paganism, Wicca, and Druidry more popular than ever, all part of a contemporary 'occulture'. According to Christopher Partridge, all of these movements share a 'background knowledge' of spiritual and mythical experience which informs their 'plausibility structures' (Partridge, 2004–2005, p. 187).

Metaphysically based practices such as these are now burgeoning exponentially and provide much needed community forums where pluralistic magical, artistic, and political expression is made possible – very much the antithesis of the split mind described throughout this chapter. The next chapter explores the tensions between science, positivism, and magical consciousness and their significance for the work of Freud and the inception of psychoanalysis.

Notes

1 This has an important relationship to Abraham and Torok's concept of 'incorporation' (1994). See Chapter 5.
2 For an in-depth exploration of these factors, please refer to Chapter 10, 'An Alien Seed: Fear and Desire in Psychotherapy'.
3 See Chapter 8 on 'culpevility' or 'the Devil's culpa'.

4 In practice, 'Greek' usually means 'Athenian'. The ' "Greeks" were actually a conglomeration of disparate societies living both in Greece itself and the islands of the Aegean, and on the western coast of what is now modern Turkey' (Maxwell-Stuart, 2017, p. 18).
5 See Chapters 3 and 4 for interpretations of Freud's work on the uncanny.

References

Baker, P. (2011). *Austin Osman Spare: The Life and Legend of London's Lost Artist*. London: Strange Attractor Press.

Bever, E. (2008). *The Realities of Witchcraft in Popular Magic in Early Modern Europe: Culture Cognition and Everyday Life*. Basingstoke and New York: Palgrave Macmillan.

Callow, J. (2018). *Embracing the Darkness*. London and New York: I.B. Tauris & Co., Ltd.

Cannon, W. B. (1942). "Voodoo" death. *American Anthropologist*, 44: 169–181 (Am J Public Health. 2002 Oct; 92(10): 1593–1596; discussion 1594–1595).

Crowley, A. (1991). *Magic in Theory and Practice*. Secaucus: Castle Books.

Davies, O. (2012). *Magic: A Very Short Introduction*. Oxford: Oxford University Press.

Ehli, B. (2017). Rationalizing Socrates' daimonion. *British Journal for the History of Philosophy*, 26(2): 225–240.

Fisher, M. (2016). *The Weird and the Eerie*. London: Repeater Books.

Frazer, J. and Fraser, R. (1994). *The Golden Bough*. Oxford: Oxford University Press.

Freud, S. (1919). The 'Uncanny'. In Freud, A., Strachey, A., Strachey, J, and Tyson A. (Eds.), *The Standard Edition of the Complete Psychological Works of Sigmund Freud, Volume XVII (1917–1919): An Infantile Neurosis and Other Works*. London: Hogarth Press and the Institute of Psychoanalysis, pp. 217–256.

Freud, S. (1960). *Totem and Taboo*. London: Routledge and Kegan Paul, Ltd.

Gager, J. G. (1992). *Curse Tablets and Binding Spells from the Ancient World*. New York: Oxford University Press.

Geller, M. J. (1997). Freud, magic and Mesopotamia: How the magic works. *Folklore*, 108(1–2): 1–7.

Grant, K. (1972). *The Magical Revival*. London: Frederick Muller.

Grant, K. (2011). Introduction. In A. O. Spare (ed), *The Book of Pleasure (Self Love): The Psychology of Ecstasy*. London: Jerusalem Press.

Greenwood, S. and Goodwyn, E. D. (2016). *Magical Consciousness: An Anthropological and Neurobiological Approach*. New York: Routledge Taylor and Francis Group.

Hutton, R. (2017). *The Witch*. New Haven: Yale University Press.

Josephson-Storm, J. A. (2017). *The Myth of Disenchantment: Magic, Modernity, and the Birth of the Human Sciences*. Chicago and London: The University of Chicago Press.

Jung, C. G. (1968). *Psychology and Alchemy* (2nd edn completely revised edn). London: Routledge & Kegan Paul, Ltd.

Kalsched, D. (1996). *The Inner World of Trauma: Archetypal Defenses of the Personal Spirit*. London: Routledge.

King, F. (1989). *Modern Ritual Magic: The Rise of Western Occultism*. Bridport: Prism Press.

Maxwell-Stuart, P. (2017). Magic in the Ancient World. In O. Davies (ed), *The Oxford Illustrated History of Magic*. Oxford: Oxford University Press, pp. 1–28.

Mistlberger, P. T. (2020). *The Dancing Sorcerer: Essays on the Mind of the Magician.* Gatineau: Anathema.

Ogden, D. (2002). *Magic, Witchcraft, and Ghosts in The Greek and Roman Worlds.* Oxford: Oxford University Press.

Ogden, T. H. (2010). On three forms of thinking: Magical thinking, dream thinking, and transformative thinking. *The Psychoanalytic Quarterly*, 79(2): 317–347.

Owen, A. (2004). *The Place of Enchantment.* Chicago: University of Chicago Press.

Page, S. (2017). Medieval Magic. In O. Davies (ed), *The Oxford Illustrated History of Magic.* Oxford: Oxford University Press, pp. 29–64.

Partridge, C. H. (2004–2005). *The Re-enchantment of the West: Alternative Spiritualities Sacralization Popular Culture and Occulture.* London: T&T Clark International.

Perera, S. (1986). *The Scapegoat Complex: Toward a Mythology of Shadow and Guilt.* Toronto: Inner City Books.

Plutarch, N., Russell, H. G., Plutarch, D. A. and Plutarch. (2010). *On the Daimonion of Socrates: Human Liberation, Divine Guidance and Philosophy.* http://deposit.d-nb.de/cgi-bin/dokserv?id=3369431&prov=M&dok_var=1&dok_ext=htm. Accessed 18/08/2022.

Russell, D. A. (2010). In N. Plutarch, H. G, Russell, D. A. Plutarch and Plutarch (eds), *On the Daimonion of Socrates: Human liberation, Divine Guidance and Philosophy.* http://deposit.d-nb.de/cgi-bin/dokserv?id=3369431&prov=M&dok_var=1&dok_ext=htm. Accessed 18/08/2022.

Seligman, K. (2018). *Mirror of Magic: A History of Magic in the Western World.* Rochester: Inner Traditions.

Spare, A. O. (2011). *The Book of Pleasure (Self Love): The Psychology of Ecstasy.* London: Jerusalem Press.

Stanley Spaeth, B. (2014). From Goddess to Hag: The Greek and the Roman Witch in Classical Literature. In K. B. Stratton and D. S. Kalleres (eds), *Daughters of Hecate: Women and Magic in the Ancient World.* Oxford: Oxford University Press.

Thomas, K. (1971). *Religion and the Decline of Magic.* London: Penguin.

Trachtenberg, J. and Idel, M. (2013). *Jewish Magic and Superstition.* Lexington: Lexington Books.

Wildon Carr, H. (2004). *Henri Bergson: The Philosophy of Change.* London: Elbiron Classics.

Williams, L. (2020). *Miracles of Our Own Making: A History of Paganism.* London: Reaktion Books.

Chapter 2

Mythopoetic Hysteria

The *Fin de Siècle*

Introduction

During the 19th/20th century *fin de siècle*, there was a burgeoning interest among the scientific and psychological community in outré psychic states such as dreams, automatism, telepathy, somnambulism, and new investigations into hypnotism and hysteria. This coincided with the magical revival; the explorations of mesmerism, animal magnetism, and spiritualism in the field of dynamic psychiatry; and the emergence of occult societies such as the Theosophical Society and the founding of the Society for Psychical Research (SPR) (Ellenberger, 1970). This chapter is an exploration of these movements, their relationships to one another, how they have impacted the psychotherapy that is practiced today, and how we think about trauma and its recovery.

C.G. Jung, whose doctoral thesis explored the occult and spiritualism, captures the essence of the *fin de siècle* age (1977c, p. 108):

> The beginning of the nineteenth century had brought us the Romantic Movement in literature, a symptom of a widespread, deep-seated longing for anything extraordinary and abnormal. People adored wallowing in Ossianic emotions, they went crazy over novels set in old castles and ruined cloisters. Everywhere prominence was given to the mystical, the hysterical; lectures about life after death, about sleepwalkers and visionaries, about animal magnetism and mesmerism, were the order of the day.

People going 'crazy over novels set in old castles' is Jung's allusion to the cultural prevalence of neo-Romantic and Gothic literature and its 'tales of divided personality, imperilled bourgeois men and sexually predatory women, haunted houses and alien invaders' which 'produced the metaphors and narrative forms through which modern selves and societies could be imagined, feared, and desired' (Burdett, 2014, p. 52). The line that Jung draws between the mythical and hysterical is also important for subsequent considerations in this chapter regarding hysteria, trauma, magical thinking, phantasy, and creativity.

DOI: 10.4324/9781003168027-3

Fin de Siècle Currents

The accusations made by the Church in the Middle Ages of a 'heretical' occult were now, in this post-Enlightenment period of the *fin de siècle*, replaced by the 'irrational' as the pejorative label *du jour*. This socio-cultural othering continued to serve an age-old means of gaining cultural currency, though it now used a different stick of orthodoxy to beat its opponents with (Boyle, 2016, p. 64). Although rigorous empiricism had now replaced saintly purity as the goal of the post-Enlightenment, it was based on equally subjective philosophical, religious, and political preoccupations which were often far from rational (Sommer, 2016; Massicotte, 2014).

Psychology was a nascent discipline in the late 19th century and needed to establish itself against the rising popularity of spiritualism, which itself harboured an increasing desire to be seen as scientifically legitimate (Luckhurst, 2002). Yet spiritualism's metaphysical foundations meant that the shadow of the occult loomed large once again and presented a fresh challenge in this era of newly enlightened consciousness (Massicotte, 2014, p. 91). Spiritualists posited that mediums were gifted with telegraphic powers, which meant that they could receive invisible spiritual communications through the ether, which was equated with the occult signals carried by electromagnetic waves, radiation, and X-rays. Inherent in the Spiritualists' analogy were the empirical foundations that 'proved' telepathy and precognition: mediums were conductors of spirits as telegraph wires were of electricity, and both were becoming increasingly abundant (Luckhurst, 2002).

Magical Invocations: Spiritualism, Theosophy, and Occult Entities

Spiritualism influenced turn-of-the-century neo-theosophists Annie Besant and Charles Leadbeater, who drew upon its use of the occult to expand considerably on the work of the co-founder of the organisation, Madame Blavatsky. Blavatsky had also been a follower of Spiritualism, yet she later discredited it. Nevertheless, she believed herself to be a medium and privately claimed that this capacity helped her to write her seminal occult text *The Secret Doctrine*, which contained the spiritual knowledge that her Indian 'masters' had transmitted (Owen, 2004; Poller, 2018). Besant and Leadbeater would, though, expand considerably on Blavatsky's occult remit into astral travel, 'occult chemistry', and the investigation of past lives and mythical civilisations such as Atlantis and Lemuria (Poller, 2018).

The means of magical invocation used by the Spiritualists and Theosophists, colloquially known today as 'channelling', which is used to receive and communicate secret knowledge, was to become central to other important occult and psychological works written in the early 20th century. Occultist Aleister Crowley used automatic writing to transcribe his 'Guardian angel' Aiwass's rapid dictation, resulting in his *Liber AL vel Legis* (*The Book of the Law*), upon which is founded the religion of Thelema. *Liber AL vel Legis* states that the Aeon of the male Egyptian deity Osiris who had superseded the female Isis is to be replaced by the Aeon of the infant god Horus, the foremost principle of which is this highly charged maxim:

> Do what thou wilt shall be the whole of the law. . . . There is no law beyond do what thou wilt. Love is the law, love under will.
> (Crowley, cited in Owen, 2004, p. 212).

Crowley becomes the anointed prophet of this Aeon as Therion, the Beast 666 (ibid.). Jung also held inner conversations with Philemon, a *daimonic* entity he encountered in a dream in 1913, documented in his posthumously published *Liber Novus* (*The Red Book*). These conversations were part of a channelling process of 'active imagination' which is recounted in his memoir *Memories Dreams and Reflections*:

> Philemon and other figures of my fantasies brought home to me the crucial insight that there are things in the psyche which I do not produce, but which produce themselves and have their own life. Philemon represented a force which was not myself.
> (Jung, 1963, p. 176)

Although Aiwass and Philemon are markedly different psychic entities, each communicates wisdom that *daimonically* manifests as independent of the psychic vessel of the chosen recipient.

Jung's formal research into the occult would begin early in his career and continue throughout his life. His 1902 paper 'On the Psychology and Pathology of Occult Phenomena' researched mediumship as part of his medical degree and uses his cousin Helene Preiswerk and seven other mediums as his case studies. Drawing on the work of Flournoy, Janet, and Myers, Jung points to the mediums' propensity to hysteria and dissociation, which would become a significant influence on his later formulations of the complexes and collective unconscious (Shamdasani, 2015, p. 297). Jung posits that the somnambulistic states of the medium lead to a 'heightened unconscious', based on an 'intuitive knowledge' which is superior to that of the conscious mind (Jung, 1977a, p. 104; Shamdasani, 2015, p. 295).

Subliminal Selves: Frederick Myers and the Society for Psychical Research

The formation of the SPR by Myers and Gurney in London in 1882 meant that extreme states of mind were now to be taken seriously. Spiritualist mediums were of great interest to SPR researchers since they seemed able to 'split consciousness' and achieve self-induced semi-somnambulistic, trance states; yet to protect its cachet of empirical legitimacy, research was couched in terms of the supernormal rather than the supernatural (Ellenberger, 1970).

The aims of the SPR were heralded as

an organised and systemic attempt to investigate the large group of debatable phenomena designated by such terms as mesmeric, psychical and spiritualistic.

(cited in Luckhurst, 2002, p. 56).

The SPR did not, however, wish to be identified with other occult organisations such as Blavatsky's Theosophical Society, into which the SPR carried out an investigation and concluded that its 'belief system' was fraudulent (Luckhurst, 2002, p. 57). Nevertheless, this new debunking of occultism was politically problematic, particularly given that Spiritualists, who had been so important in the foundation of the SPR, refused to buy into the supernormal paradigm, thereby creating a schism within the organisation (Luckhurst, 2002; Massicotte, 2014).

By the end of the 19th century, Frederic Myers had become a respected psychologist and, in 1888, became the SPR's leading theorist. His research interests were broad, covering science, theology, metaphysics, and psychology. His research to some extent mirrored the investigations of those of the *fin de siècle* such as Charcot, Freud, Janet, and Jung. Myers researched the 'hypnoid states' of dissociated personality, hypnagogia, and telepathy, all of which would inform his theory of the 'subliminal self' (Luckhurst, 2002; Taves, 2003). Myers's meta-psychology not only contains a 'subliminal' unconscious self but also one which transcends the 'supraliminal' (a rather utilitarian, conscious self). As it is modelled on a spectrum of psychic life based on the evolutionary theories of the physical sciences, Myers's self extends 'down' to the automatic physiological layers of the subconscious (including what is now known as 'procedural' or 'implicit' memory), yet the subliminal self has the capacity to evolve 'up' to higher states of consciousness, where the subject has the potential to access clairvoyant, telepathic levels of consciousness (Luckhurst, 2002, p. 109).

The lack of 'primacy' of Myers's waking self and the postulation of unconscious affects, thoughts, and memories at the time drew comparisons with Freud's unconscious and Janet's 'secondary selves', though an important distinction was made by Freud himself in his first paper published to an English-speaking readership in 1912, *A Note on the Unconscious*. Freud would become a corresponding member of the SPR from 1911 until 1938, and the publication of his monograph served to begin an important process of distinction from the work of Myers; Charcot; and his main rival, Janet (Gyimesi, 2009; Keeley, 2001; Massicotte, 2014). Freud used this opportunity to make it clear that his dynamic unconscious does not contain 'parts' of a personality that can be integrated, unlike Myers's model, which indicates potential unity. The Freudian unconscious works in opposition to its conscious counterpart, and for Freud, things don't ascend any 'higher' than the conscious mind (Gyimesi, 2009; Keeley, 2001; Luckhurst, 2002; Taves, 2003). Yet despite Freud's clear distinction – in keeping with his uncomfortable ambivalence regarding the occult that will become clearer – he somewhat paradoxically makes complementary reference to the work of Carl du Prel and his 'transcendent self' in *The Interpretation of Dreams*. Du Prel's subjectivity ascends *beyond* the functions of the waking self and in this way bears some similarity to Myers's own formulation (Boyle, 2016).

In terms of the clinical material to be examined in later chapters, Myers is undoubtedly an important yet largely forgotten figure in early trauma research due to his concept of the 'multiplex' personality, now referred to as dissociative identities and the development of magical consciousness (Taves, 2003). Myers saw evidence of these split-off parts of the personality acting independently of the subject's conscious ego (Luckhurst, 2002; Taves, 2003). Myers also coined the concept of telepathy, or 'the communication of any impressions of any kind from one mind to another, independently of the recognised channels of sense' (cited in Luckhurst, 2002, p. 113).

The SPR's interest in telepathy resulted in the foundation of a dedicated research committee. Its objective was for its telepathic experiments to become recognised by the scientific community and become its very own 'black box', thereby distinguishing itself from Spiritualism (Luckhurst, 2002, p, 70). However, due to the revelation that its research subjects had sent coded messages to one another, this was soon discredited. Yet research into telepathy was very much concordant with the preoccupations of physicists of the time, whose research into transmissions through electromagnetic rays and radio waves provided the SPR with new impetus to find fresh evidence of its mechanisms (Luckhurst, 2002).

Somewhat ironically, the SPR shared the same strategy as the Spiritualists they had discredited by pointing to telegraphic communications as evidence of the possibility of thought transference. Psychic phenomena apparent at séances attributed by Spiritualists to the communications of the dead were, for Myers and colleagues, interpreted as communications by the 'subliminal self' (ibid.). For Myers and the SPR, telepathy becomes the crown jewel of a hermeneutics of the unconscious, though importantly within the model of the 'subliminal self', telepathy explains both intra- and intersubjective unconscious and conscious processes. However, the (unconscious) 'subliminal self' was not always a reliable narrator to the (conscious) 'supraliminal self', and messages may be corrupted when crossing the threshold of consciousness, thereby explaining the fragmentary alters of mediums and the dissociative states of hysteria (Ko, 2007, p. 744). Importantly, Frederick Myers does not equate hysteria only with psychopathology, noting that the porous nature of the hysterical subliminal self explains genius and contains an unconscious 'mythopoetic' function which includes fantasies and the seeds of creativity (Ellenberger, 1970, p. 355). Myers therefore recognises the difference between magical thinking and consciousness.

Black Tides: Psychoanalysis and the Occult

The generally received opinion regarding Freud and the occult is that he was part of a highly rationalist, Darwinian materialism that ranged from indifference to hostility to the supernatural. However, his paper *Psychoanalysis and Telepathy*, presented to a select group of colleagues in 1921, conveys a cautious, open-minded and sympathetic attitude.

> It does not follow as a matter of course that an intensified interest in occultism must involve a danger to psycho-analysis. We should, on the contrary, be prepared to find reciprocal sympathy between them. They have both experienced the same contemptuous and arrogant treatment by official science. To this day psycho-analysis is regarded as savouring of mysticism, and its unconscious is looked upon as one of the things between heaven and earth which philosophy refuses to dream of.
>
> (Freud, 1941 [1921], p. 178)

Despite Freud's apparent rapprochement with occultists, he knew that for psychoanalysis to be accepted as a science, he would need to distance his own discipline from esotericism, and it would be his libido theory which became the key demarcating function (Gyimesi, 2009). This perspective accounts for Freud's vehement attack on Jung when he challenged the older man on the necessity of libido theory and put forward his theory of the collective unconscious, both tantamount to letting in a 'black tide of mud' (Jung, 1963, pp. 147–148; Richardson, 2018). Paradoxically, in 1921, Freud wrote to the psychical researcher Hereward Carrington,

> I am not one of those who dismiss a priori the study of so-called occult psychic phenomena as unscientific, discreditable or even as dangerous. If I were at the beginning rather than at the end of a scientific career, as I am today, I might possibly choose just this field of research, in spite of all difficulties.
>
> (quoted in Gyimesi, 2009, p. 463)

Freud would subsequently repudiate this statement and in the same year write of occultists,

> the faith which they first adopt themselves and then seek to impose on other people is either the old religious faith which has been pushed into the background by science in the course of human development, or another one even closer to the superseded convictions of primitive peoples. Analysts, on the other hand, cannot repudiate their descent from exact science and their community with its representatives. . . . The analyst has his own province of work, which he must not abandon: the unconscious element of mental life.
>
> (Freud, 1941 [1921], pp. 178–179)

Here, Freud returns to the Frazerian hypothesis of equating 'primitive' magical thinking with developmental arrest. This pejorative idea of the 'primitive' contrasts with that of Jung, who holds up 'primitive man' as a source of inspiration, as his dreams hold greater value for him than his 'civilised' counterpart (1977b, p. 130). The *fin de siècle* author Arthur Machen goes even further, locating the 'miraculous' in the child and primitive man – the most desirable, ecstatic state of consciousness (1926, p. 176). Elsewhere, Freud endearingly expresses a humble awareness towards the allure of the 'miraculous mind' in himself as much as others:

> If one regards oneself as a sceptic, it is a good plan to have occasional doubts about one's scepticism too. It may be that I too have a secret inclination towards the miraculous which thus goes half way to meet the creation of occult facts.
>
> (Freud, 1933 [1932], p. 53)

Freud therefore appears to struggle between maintaining the safely moored legitimacy of the sceptical materialist and his own predilection for the 'miraculous'. Nevertheless, the tensions and anxieties evident in Freud's writing on the occult, which were to no small extent provoked by a jostling among several different movements to claim an authoritative epistemology of the mind, provided fertile ground for the early psychoanalytic movement to emerge (Gyimesi, 2009; Massicotte, 2014; Richardson, 2018).

At the time of the foundation of the British Psychoanalytical Society in 1919 and the *International Journal of Psychoanalysis* in 1920, as a result of the fervent campaigns of Ernest Jones, psychoanalysis was on the brink of being accepted into the medical and scientific establishments (Richardson, 2018, p. 115). However, its practitioners, who comprised both medical professionals and lay analysts, were more diverse in terms of their modality and the barriers between a materialist and metaphysical *weltanschauung*, were porous (Richardson, 2018, p. 115).

The first institution to provide psychoanalytic instruction in Britain was London's Medico-Psychological Clinic in Brunswick Square. Here, candidates would receive instruction in psychoanalysis alongside electrotherapy, hypnosis, and suggestion (ibid.). Violet Firth, now better known as the occultist and writer Dion Fortune, trained as a lay analyst at the clinic and subsequently founded her own occult society, the Fraternity of the Inner Light. Fortune valued Freud's work on the unconscious and returned his 'reciprocal sympathy' by recommending that her esoteric students read *The Interpretation of Dreams* (Boyle, 2016). The philosophy of the Kabbalah would become an important influence on her occult work, leading to the publication of her much cited esoteric text *Mystical Qabalah*, and here Fortune provides another, perhaps unexpected, link with Freud who was – various scholars claim – through his family's Jewish and Hasidic heritage, also influenced by the Kabbalah (Schneider and Berke, 2008; Boyle, 2016). Schneider and Berke draw parallels between the secret, hidden worlds of the Kabbalah and the psychoanalytic unconscious, as well as their relationship to an external reality which folds back in on itself, thereby also finding links with Klein's paradigm of introjection and projection (2008).

From Wishes to Clairvoyance: Psychoanalysis and Telepathy

Despite Jung's objections, libido theory and the dynamic unconscious would become important cornerstones of Freudian theory and would enable Freud to differentiate his work from Spiritualism and from rivals such as Janet and Myers. Nevertheless, Freud shared his rivals' desire to find a satisfactory hermeneutic system for phenomena where material explanations fell short, and it was in thought transference, more commonly known as telepathy, that he saw a 'kernel of truth' (Jones, in Massicotte, 2014).

In *Dreams and Occultism*, Freud makes his contempt towards séance mediums clear, asserting that their 'performances give one the impression of children's mischievous pranks or conjuring tricks' (Freud, 1933 [1932], p. 35). Yet it seems he may have been reserving his scorn for the sleight of hand that had given the séance a bad reputation, as in the same paper – although outrightly dismissing any possibility of mediums' precognitive skills – he attributes some competence to their telepathic abilities: after attending a séance held by the medium Frau Seidler with Ferenczi in 1909, Freud equivocally states that Seidler had been able to read Ferenczi's mind (Massicotte, 2014, p. 96).

Freud highlights the importance of affect in telepathy, though he also scornfully refers to the 'sensitive' capacity attributed to the séance mediums (1933 [1932], p. 36). After carrying out telepathic experiments with both Ferenczi and Anna Freud, Freud then concludes that his daughter possesses a 'telepathic sensitivity' (quoted in Rabeyron and Evrard, 2012, p. 13). Freud's emphasis on this emotional component of thought transference therefore parallels Jung's and Myers's equation of mediumship with the 'sensitivity' of hysteria.

In *Psychoanalysis and Telepathy*, Freud presents the case of a man who visits a fortune teller who predicts that his brother-in-law will die of crayfish or oyster poisoning (1941 [1921]). The prophesy comes true to some extent in that he is indeed poisoned by crayfish, though he survives. Freud again dismisses any possibility of precognition and interprets this in Oedipal terms: the medium is merely responding to his client's wish to kill his brother-in-law. Importantly, however, the wish was still transmitted unconsciously – or telepathically – and in *Dreams and Occultism* more than ten years later, Freud strongly indicates his belief in telepathic communication:

> I must confess that I have a feeling that here too the scale weights in favor of thought-transference.
>
> (1933 [1932], p. 54)

In the same paper, Freud presents a case of a woman who visits a medium who predicts that she will have two children by the age of 32; the same age her mother had been when she gave birth to her two children (Freud, 1933 [1932]). When the woman visits Freud as a patient in her early forties, remaining childless, he interprets that the medium had unconsciously responded to the patient's wish to take her mother's place, as evidenced by the numbers two and 32. With this example, Freud once again emphasises the potency of unconscious wishes.

In *Psychoanalysis and Telepathy*, Freud notes the medium's

> function of diverting her own psychical forces and occupying them in a harmless way, so that she could become receptive and accessible to the effects upon her of her client's thoughts.
>
> (Freud, 1941 [1921])

The medium's skill that Freud highlights calls to mind his recommended technique of 'evenly suspended attention' for psychoanalysts in his paper on recommended technique (Freud, 1912, p. 115). Freud stipulates that the analyst

> must turn his own unconscious like a receptive organ towards the transmitting unconscious of the patient.

The analyst here then essentially *becomes a medium* to his patient, yet unlike the clairvoyant, who is 'accessible to her client's thoughts upon her', the analyst must also be like 'a surgeon, who puts aside all his feelings' (ibid.). Therefore, although the analyst uses the unconscious as a 'receptor', it is to be used only as an *instrument* and should not therefore become prey to the distortions which lead to the wish-fulfilment–generated enactments of the examples above. There are implicit stereotypes here which, of course, are of their time: the hysterical, emotional (female) medium versus the forensic, objective (male) surgeon.

Becoming a Medium: Sandor Ferenczi

With Sandor Ferenczi's work, psychoanalysis takes its first relational turn. For Ferenczi, the psychoanalyst is not merely a neutral, objective instrument. Instead, the analyst *becomes* a medium for the unbearable feelings and thoughts of the patient (Phillips, cited in Farber, 2017, p. 722). Nevertheless, the idea of psychoanalysts *becoming* mediums was out of the question for Freud: although he had encouraged Ferenczi in his research into thought transference, he also urged caution in this regard (Massicotte, 2014). Telepathy's association with the occult meant it presented a threat to the 'demarcating' element of libido theory which, for Freud, was the key to being accepted within the scientific orthodoxy (Gyimesi, 2009, p. 460).

Despite Ferenczi's interest in telepathy, his own approach remained scientific, which to some extent parallels the work of the SPR. However, there is an added innovative, intuitive element to his clinical work. Like Freud, Ferenczi understood the power of influence of affect in relation to thought transference/telepathy, but his additional interest lay in exploring the way in which these elements interact with one another and impact upon processes of transference and countertransference. The consulting room for Ferenczi therefore becomes an arena where telepathy and transference continually converge and *haunt* psychoanalysis (Gyimesi, 2012; Luckhurst, 2002, p. 75). The transference situation therefore awakens a telepathic sensitivity in the patient, which in traumatised individuals can reach a 'clairvoyant' level:

> Whether they recognize the truth by the intonation or colour of our voice or by the words we use or in some other way, I cannot tell. In any case, they show a remarkable, almost clairvoyant knowledge about the thoughts and emotions that go on in their analyst's mind.
>
> (Ferenczi, 1988, p. 200).

In Ferenczi's work – and as with Freud, Jung, and Myers – there is to varying degrees an equation between the 'sensitive' yet fragmented mind of the medium and the hysterical/traumatised patient whose only recourse is to split or dissociate. Yet to some degree, Ferenczi himself was able to, if not heal the split between psychoanalysis and the occult, at least use the language of the latter to alchemically forge a new clinical epistemology of relational and intrapsychic trauma which has seen a renaissance in recent years. Beyond the application of Ferenczi's occult research and his clinical work on trauma and its dissociative defences, we also see a very important legacy in terms of thinking about their relevance to transferential processes in the consulting room, encompassing countertransference, introjection, and projection and the concept of projective identification, the last of these formulated by Ferenczi's former patient Melanie Klein. These aspects of Ferenczi's work are explored in further detail in Chapter 6.

Concluding Discussion

This chapter illustrates the importance of the visionary movements of psychology, science, and the occult during the *fin de siècle* and, as with the previous chapter, a need to 'demarcate' in order to conform to socio-cultural orthodoxies, yet for psychoanalysis, it was due to potential accusations of irrationality rather than apostasy. As has become apparent, metaphysical epistemologies which may appear to be confined to the fringes also find themselves very much at home in psychotherapy, even if these roots are not commonly acknowledged: in contemporary psychotherapies, one can see the influence of the *fin de siècle* research of the Theosophists in past life regression and family constellations therapies, both of which to differing extents posit that intergenerational experiences can be accessed either through hypnosis or through group work, respectively. Due to these occult associations, both therapies may appear to operate on the outer limits, but the sheer number of practitioners offering their services online suggests otherwise. This highlights the deficit in material approaches, which confine clients to an individual body and implicitly minimise transcendent and transpersonal experiences of magical consciousness.

The influence of Madame Blavatsky's pioneering imbrication of Eastern mysticism and Western esotericism can be found in other, less 'transcendent' Western psychotherapy approaches today. The health benefits of yoga and meditation are now widely accepted in the mainstream, though during the *fin de siècle*, this kind of heterodoxy was still considered radical. The Theosophists' merging of East and West is also found in psychotherapies which focus on treating trauma and advocate the clinical use of Eastern spiritual disciplines such as yoga and mindfulness practices. There are also echoes of occult currents in internal family systems therapy, gestalt psychotherapy, transactional analysis, and Jungian analysis, where to varying degrees there are separate 'parts' of the personality which have, to varied extents, independent agency. These entities may be malignant or benevolent, but there is a common idea that they hold a wisdom that the individual should take note of, and the psychotherapist helps the client to engage these 'selves' into a dialogue facilitated by means of invocation such as meditative exercises, art making, visualisation, or role play. Both Crowley's and Jung's means of engaging their own hitherto unknown selves were also forms of magical invocation, and various interpretations of Jung's 'active imagination' are seen in psychotherapy consulting rooms today as inroads into the unconscious (Singer, 1994). If these clinical invocations are to be successful, some level of relaxation is required in order for the other parts of the personality to be engaged by a central ego and are, therefore, to some extent analogous with the trance states required in mediumship and artificially induced hypnosis. It is important to note that these clinical theories are predicated on the idea that in psychopathology and trauma, the mind is split and dissociative rather than the repressive, dynamic unconscious of psychoanalysis and therefore maintains the 'demarcation' between Janet/Myers/Jung and Freud in contemporary psychotherapy. Nonetheless, Jung, Freud, Janet, Myers, and most notably Ferenczi share the view that mediums possess a heightened *sensitivity* which explains both their capacity for hysteria but also for telepathy and clairvoyance.

Hysteria today is now much more commonly framed in a paradigm of trauma, yet it is Ferenczi's pioneering research and compassionate sensitivity which led him to think about this convergence between the hysterical/traumatised patient and the medium in terms of the 'clairvoyant' child who develops a sixth sense as a means of identifying with and defending against an abusive caregiver. Myers and Jung go further and link this clairvoyant sensitivity not only to the traumatised individual's capacity for telepathy but also to the heightened intelligence of their unconscious and its significant mythopoetic function (Ellenberger, 1970, p. 788; Jung, 1977a, p. 104). These mythopoetic, clairvoyant capacities are often evident in traumatised individuals whose heightened sensitivity combines with a notably imaginative and creative mind. If this imaginative capacity can be harnessed positively, and a positive transference achieved by careful attention to the implicit relational aspects of the therapeutic relationship, this presents an opportunity for pathological phantasies and identifications to be worked through and can help clients move out of painful self-object repetition compulsions towards more harmonious relational experiences. However, as will become clear in subsequent chapters, this is far from guaranteed and requires significant work and patience on the part of the psychotherapist. These dissociative defences, phantasies, and identifications of the traumatised self and their relation to the mythopoetic experiences of magical consciousness are also all-important aspects which concern the 'curse position' set out in the following chapter.

References

Boyle, J. (2016). Esoteric traces in contemporary psychoanalysis. *American Imago*, 73(1): 95–119.

Burdett, C. (2014). Modernity, the Occult and Psychoanalysis'. In L. Marcus and A. Mukhurjee (eds), *A Concise Companion to Psychoanalysis, Literature, and Culture*. Hoboken: Wiley and Sons, pp. 49–65.

Ellenberger, H. F. (1970). *The Discovery of the Unconscious; The History and Evolution of Dynamic Psychiatry*. New York: Basic Books.

Farber, S. K. (2017). Becoming a telepathic tuning fork: Anomalous experience and the relational mind. *Psychoanalytic Dialogues*, 27(6): 719–734.

Ferenczi, S. (1988). Confusion of tongues between adults and the child: The language of tenderness and of passion. *Contemporary Psychoanalysis*, 24(2): 196–206.

Freud, S. (1912). Recommendations to Physicians Practising Psychoanalysis. In Freud, A., Strachey, A., Strachey, J, and Tyson A. (Eds.), *The Standard Edition of the Complete Psychological Works of Sigmund Freud, Volume XII (1911–1913): The Case of Schreber, Papers on Technique and Other Works*. London: Hogarth Press and the Institute of Psychoanalysis, pp. 109–120.

Freud, S. (1941 [1921]). Psycho-Analysis and Telepathy. In Freud, A., Strachey, A., Strachey, J, and Tyson A. (Eds.), *The Standard Edition of the Complete Psychological Works of Sigmund Freud, Volume XVIII (1920–1922): Beyond the Pleasure Principle, Group Psychology and Other Works*. London: Hogarth Press and the Institute of Psychoanalysis, pp. 173–194.

Freud, S. (1933 [1932]). Dreams and Occultism. In Freud, A., Strachey, A., Strachey, J, and Tyson A. (Eds.), *The Standard Edition of the Complete Psychological Works of Sigmund Freud, Volume XXII (1932–1936): New Introductory Lectures on Psycho-Analysis and Other Works*. London: The Hogarth Press and the Institute of Psycho-analysis, pp. 1–267.

Gyimesi, J. (2009). The problem of demarcation: Psychoanalysis and the occult. *American Imago*, 66(4): 457–470.

Gyimesi, J. (2012). Sándor Ferenczi and the problem of telepathy. *History of the Human Sciences*, 25(2): 131–148.

Jung, C. G. (1977a). On the Psychology of So-Called Occult Phenomena. In *Psychology and the Occult*. Princeton: Princeton University Press, pp. 4–106.

Jung, C. G. (1977b). The Psychological Foundations of Belief in Spirits. In *Psychology and the Occult*. Princeton: Princeton University Press, pp. 129–148.

Jung, C. G. (1977c). On Spiritualistic Phenomena. In *Psychology and the Occult*. Princeton: Princeton University Press, pp. 106–126.

Jung, C. G. and Jaffé, A. (1963). *Memories, Dreams, Reflections*. London: Collins, Routledge and Kegan Paul.

Keeley, J. P. (2001). Subliminal promptings: Psychoanalytic theory and the society for psychical research. *American Imago*, 58(4): 767–791.

Ko, C. (2007). Subliminal consciousness. *The Review of English Studies*, 59(242): 740–765.

Luckhurst, R. (2002). *The Invention of Telepathy, 1870–1901*. Oxford: Oxford University Press.

Machen, A. (1926). *Hieroglyphics*. London: Martin Secker.

Massicotte, C. (2014). Psychical transmissions: Freud, spiritualism, and the occult. *Psychoanalytic Dialogues*, 24(1): 88–102.

Owen, A. (2004). *The Place of Enchantment*. Chicago: University of Chicago Press.

Poller, J. (2018). Under a Glamour: Annie Besant, Charles Leadbeater and Neo-theosophy. In C. Ferguson and Radford (eds), *The Occult Imagination in Britain*. London and New York: Routledge, pp. 77–93.

Rabeyron, T. and Evrard, R. (2012). Historical and contemporary perspectives on occultism in the Freud-Ferenczi correspondence. *Recherches en Psychanalyse*, 13(1): 98–111.

Richardson, E. (2018). Stemming the Black Tide of Mud. In C. Ferguson and Radford (eds), *The Occult Imagination in Britain*. London and New York: Routledge, pp. 110–128.

Schneider, S. and Berke, J. H. (2008). The oceanic feeling, Mysticism and Kabbalah: Freud's historical roots. *The Psychoanalytic Review*, 95(1): 131–156.

Shamdasani, S. (2015). "S.W." and C.G. Jung: Mediumship, psychiatry and serial exemplarity. *History of Psychiatry*, 26(3): 288–302.

Singer, J. (1994). *Boundaries of the Soul*. Garden City: Anchor, Doubleday.

Sommer, A. (2016). Are you afraid of the dark? Notes on the psychology of belief in histories of science and the occult. *European Journal of Psychotherapy & Counselling*, 18(2): 105–122.

Taves, A. (2003). Religious experience and the divisible self: William James (and Frederic Myers) as theorist(s) of religion. *Journal of the American Academy of Religion*, 71(2): 303–326.

Chapter 3

The Curse Position (1)

Unconscious Phantasy

Introduction

As we have seen in Chapter 1, attributing the uncanny nature of misfortune to random chance alone is often insufficient: people generally wish to attribute bad luck
to 'human or superhuman' agencies (Hutton, 2017, p. 10). In the 'curse position',
this sense of misfortune becomes 'uncanny', as it is both disturbing yet familiar:
it underpins one's identity, rendering the individual spellbound. This position is
returned to repetitively, and the individual is at the mercy of painful affective experiences of self-object sabotage.

This chapter explores unconscious phantasy in terms of its relationship to the
curse position. I provide an overview of differing perspectives on unconscious
phantasy which are relevant to the curse position and clinical work. I then set
out essential elements of the curse position. I subsequently highlight potent and
charged psychic phenomena which stem from the archaic unconscious and how
they impact upon the aetiology of curse position and its related unconscious
phantasies. I then present a basic theory of mind of the curse position: The 'curse'
is subdivided into two levels of interdependent psychic experience: the 'primary
curse' consists of unconscious phantasy and the fear based sequelae of the archaic unconscious. The subject attempts to make sense of and symbolise these
overwhelmingly persecutory elements but ultimately fails to do so, and this then
becomes a 'secondary curse'.

The persecutory influence of this archaic, deeper unconscious is illustrated by
the M.R. James short story 'Oh, Whistle and I'll Come to You, My Lad'. The chapter ends with a case illustration as an example of the presented theories in clinical
practice.

A Note on Terminology

In this chapter and throughout this book, I will be using *phantasy* to refer to the
psychoanalytic concept of unconscious phantasy and reserve *fantasy* for its more
colloquial use: of dreaming about or imagining.

DOI: 10.4324/9781003168027-4

Phantasy: An Overview

I now provide a non-exhaustive overview of the different psychoanalytic perspectives of unconscious phantasy that have developed over the years, through to the present day.

Studies in Hysteria features Breuer and Freud earliest formulations on phantasy, though they do not specifically use the term (2004). Their focus at this point is on the split, dissociative mind of hysteria with its tendency towards daydreams:

> These hypnoid states, however varied they may be, have one thing in common with each other and with hypnosis, notably that the ideas within them are very intense, but are blocked from associative exchange with the remaining element of consciousness.

> (2004, p. 15)

Freud and Breuer postulate that 'hypnoid states' stem from the 'daydreams' of 'healthy people', though in order to illustrate the psychopathological aspects of phantasy, they draw a parallel between the psychotic element of dreams and hypnoid states, where the former are benignly contained in sleep, and the latter may 'jut over in waking life in the form of hysterical phenomena' (Breuer and Freud, 2004, p. 16). Here, Freud and Breuer therefore make the distinction between daydream/pre-conscious fantasies and unconscious phantasies.

For Freud, phantasy played a significant part in terms of his abandonment of 'seduction theory'. The causative emphasis for hysterical psychopathology therefore shifted from actual events of childhood sexual abuse to the blocking of the subject's wishes, forming his topographical model (Bohleber et al., 2015; Laplanche and Pontalis, 1973; Spillius, 2001). This formation of phantasy as the blocking and frustration of the drive is what Spillius calls Freud's 'central usage' (Spillius, 2001).

In his 1908 paper *Hysterical Phantasies and Their Relation to Bisexuality*, Freud states:

> Unconscious phantasies are either those that have always been unconscious and were formed in the unconscious or, as is more frequently the case, those that were once conscious phantasies, daydreams which have then deliberately been forgotten and got into the unconscious through 'repression'.

> (2004, p. 310)

Here, Freud distinguishes between inherited phylogenetic memories – those that have always been unconscious – and the 'central usage' stemming from secondary process and repression.

Melanie Klein radically alters the concept of unconscious phantasy, as adumbrated in Susan Isaac's seminal 1948 paper *The Nature and Function of Phantasy*, which played a significant part in the 'controversial discussions' of the British

Psychoanalytic Society. Based on Klein's analysis of infant play in the first three years of life, unconscious phantasy becomes all encompassing: it is not only the mental manifestation of the biological instincts but also the 'primary content of all unconscious processes' (Isaacs, 1948, p. 80). For Isaacs, unconscious phantasy is also the representative of all bodily processes and affects, their satisfactions, and frustrations: it is *our hallucinations of them which help us to anticipate and represent reality* (Isaacs, 1948, p. 90; italics my own). Klein herself also emphasises this 'hallucinatory' aspect of phantasy and its impact on object relations:

> In hallucinatory gratification, therefore, two unrelated processes take place; the omnipotent conjuring up of the ideal object and situation, and the equally omnipotent annihilation of the bad persecutory object and the painful situation.
>
> (Klein, 1946, p. 7)

Klein and her followers have faced some criticism over the years, as their version of unconscious phantasy is an *a priori* psychic reality which would involve a sophisticated level of mental functioning that Piaget's research has shown to be impossible, in addition to the fact that its permeation of all psychic processes potentially renders it meaningless (Bohleber et al., 2015, p. 709; Ogden, 1984, p. 501). In the 1960s, Kleinian unconscious phantasy expanded to incorporate intersubjective phenomena using the model of gestalt field psychology to explain co-created phantasies and projective identifications. This goes some way to further account for the mystical, quasi-telepathic evolutions of projective identification that are discussed in Chapter 10 (Bohleber et al., 2015, p. 708).

Much has been made by Kleinians of the relationship between phantasy, creativity, and play, with the latter becoming a vehicle to explore phantasies in the presence of the therapist (Isaacs, 1948; Segal, 1994). Yet it is Winnicott who audaciously shifts play away from the Kleinian pathologies of endogenous phantasy towards a two-person psychology, where it becomes part of a 'facilitating environment' (1965, p. 85). According to Winnicott, where there are failures in the facilitating environment, children retreat to 'fantasying', a pathogenic form of dissociation where the individual is neither dreaming nor living (Winnicott, 1982, p. 36; Davies and Frawley, 1992).

With the emergence of Bowlby's attachment theory, there is a further shift towards outside world experience. Unconscious phantasy is now replaced by 'internal working models', emphasising 'veridical' experience (Erreich, 2015, p. 2). Daniel Stern's clinical research has been instrumental in terms of integrating Bowlby's work with object relations, libido theory, and cognitive science. Stern postulates that unconscious phantasy is part of a 'pre-narrative envelope' which includes

> instinctual urgings, visual images, affect shifts, sensations, motor actions, ideas, states of arousal, language, place, space time, etc.
>
> (Stern, 1992, p. 295)

All of these processes are unconscious, of which drives and wishes are a part, but not the totality; in their 'pandemonium', they form an 'emergent property of mind' which integrates all of these experiences (ibid.). Anne Erreich continues along Stern's line of perceiving phantasy as the totality of a diverse range of representational processes including both the perceptions of the veridical interpersonal experiences of the subject as well as her intra-psychic conflicts and defences (Erreich, 2015). Hewitt importantly emphasises the way in which internal representations of 'emotional states' and the capacity to reflect upon them can be impinged upon by the distortions of unconscious phantasy and trauma (2020, p. 20).

The Curse Position: An Overview

Before setting out the relationship between unconscious phantasy and the curse position, I now set out the core elements of the latter.

As stated in the Introduction, I could not have developed the theory of the curse position without Freud's *The Uncanny* and Mark Fisher's *The Weird and the Eerie*. Freud defines *The Uncanny* as

> that class of the terrifying which leads back to something long known to us, once very familiar.
>
> (1919, p. 220)

It is what reveals itself yet what we feel should not which creates a familiarity between what is *heimlich* (homely), and *unheimlich* (unhomely).[1] The uncanny nature of the curse position renders the homely unhomely and vice versa; self-object representations are ruptured by trauma and then bound by unconscious phantasy. These phantasies create images and disturbing affects that are familiar (*heimlich*) yet may be experienced as hostile (*unheimlich*) substitutes. Mark Fisher's *The Weird and the Eerie*, published almost 100 years after Freud's *The Uncanny*, offers new perspectives on uncanny experience in relation to trauma and, therefore, to the phenomenology of the curse position. According to Fisher, the uncanny experience is to view the outside from the inside (though an outside which can never fully be acknowledged), whereas the 'weird' and the 'eerie' perform the opposite function (2016, p. 10).[2] The 'weird' concerns *presence* of '*that which does not belong*' and is typified by 'the conjoining of *two or more things which do not belong together*' (Fisher, 2016, pp. 10–11). The 'eerie' concerns failures of both presence and absence (Fisher, 2016, p. 61).

> The sensation of the eerie occurs either when there is something present where there should be nothing, or there is nothing present where there should be something.
>
> (ibid.)

The curse is 'something where there should be nothing': it is *weird*, as it is experienced as alien to the individual, yet it remains *eerily* familiar (Fisher, 2016,

p. 67). These uncanny dissonances between the inside and outside, trauma and unconscious phantasy, are themselves all instrumental aspects of the subjective experience of the curse position. Fisher's work on the tensions between outside/inside and presence/absence become more pertinent clinically when we consider them alongside Winnicott's developmental paradigm and the relationship he delineates between such tensions and developmental trauma.

> It will be appreciated that this theory includes the idea of trauma, by which I mean an experience against which the ego defences were inadequate at the stage of emotional development of the individual at the time, or in the state of the patient at the time. Trauma is an impingement from the environment and from the individual's reaction to the impingement that occurs prior to the individual's development of the mechanisms that make the unpredictable predictable.
>
> (Winnicott, 2018, p. 198)

Thus, where there is a failure of the defences (failed presence), the intrusion of the unexpected (impingement – failure of absence) into the expectant familiarity of the subject's inner world, this creates a traumatic wound. Weiss highlights this conflict:

> The patient finds it difficult to think presence in the absence or to bear absence in the presence.
>
> (2021, p. 758)

These traumatising processes and the subject's reactions to them are consequently experienced as an intrusive attack on the self. As a result of these traumatic wounds, the individual begins to over-identify with a phantasy of a faulty and obsolete internal object which leads to repetitive self-sabotaging experiences which become uncannily familiar, yet – as with the experience of the original trauma – feel entirely beyond one's control. With traumatic impingement – and abandonments – caused by 'eerie' failures of absence and presence (and here I incorporate veridical experience and phantasy) there is an impact on the *agency* of the individual and one's perception of space and time (Fisher, 2016, p. 63). In terms of space, the internal agency of containing function is impaired by pathological forms of unconscious phantasy. The subject therefore resorts to seeking agency *outside the self*, though it is masochistically sought from an object which is either experienced as abandoning or impinging, thereby re-creating the original trauma.

In terms of temporal experience, the curse position is wired to an anxious preoccupation with fate: past events become future omens, which creates a 'fatalistic eternity' from which the individual cannot escape (Fisher, 2014, p. 36):

> The present tense – or rather the hesitation between past and present tense – creates an ambiguity, suggesting a fatalistic eternity, a compulsion to repeat – a

compulsion that *might* be a self-fulfilling prophecy. The ghosts return because he fears they will. . . .

(ibid.)

The subject consequently yearns for a real without fear, to which the closest she finds are moments of 'eerie calm' where the unwanted presence of mental pain is never far away (Fisher, 2016, p. 13). As Fisher points out, by drawing on medieval witch-lore, Shakespeare's *Macbeth* binds the 'weird' (lack of belonging) to '*wyrd*' (fate). The former term has evolved from the latter's Germanic etymological root. The three *wyrd* sisters, or fates, of *Macbeth* are so called as they can predict Macbeth's fate, yet an imprecation lies inside their prophecy which seals the doomed king's self-destruction. The curse therefore lies at the intersection between these two signifiers, and their conjunction sustains the 'fatalistic eternity' of the curse.

Unconscious Phantasy and the Formation of the Curse Position

Fate is experienced as eternal, in part due to its connection with forgotten aspects of one's past, particularly those from infancy. It is therefore essential to examine the influence of developmental factors on the curse position with particular regard to unconscious phantasy.

We are unable to account for much of our experience in the first three years of life, yet self-object representations are formed early on. Infant research has demonstrated that proto-representations begin as early as the first year of life (Beebe and Lachmann, 1988; Stern, 1994). At this crucial stage of development, networks of experiences begin to form early phantasies. These are representations of images, affects, and sounds, and in cases of developmental and relational trauma, this may well therefore contribute to the formation of a cursed identity. The individual then begins to feel inherently victimised, and each time she has experiences which contain the echoes of these pre-narrative events, they are felt as intrusions on her subjectivity and start to become *all too familiar* to her. Although she dissociates her traumatic memories, she is still tragically bound to identify with them. At the most extreme levels of trauma, one becomes exiled in an *abject* real where one's 'very existence is forfeited', such as in severe cases of psychopathology such as anorexia nervosa or even suicide (Kristeva, 1982, p. 9).

Unconscious phantasy and early developmental experiences are not only principal factors in identity formation but also in their relation to time and the subject's concomitant perception of fate. Developmental research has helped us to examine the temporal nature of the mother–infant dyad more closely. Both live in a 'split second world' where mutual affect regulation is influenced by the attuned temporal matching in the dyad. This forms the basis of identifications, phantasies, and – perhaps most importantly for the curse position and its relationship to fate – predictions about the future (Stern, 1994; Beebe and Lachmann, 1988).

> We suggest that, prior to the development of symbolic capacities, the infant is able to represent expected, characteristic interaction structures, including their distinctive temporal, spatial, and affective features. Toward the end of the first year, *representations of expected interaction* structures are abstracted into generalized prototypes. These generalized prototypes become the basis for later symbolic forms of self-and object representations.
>
> (Beebe and Lachmann, 1988, p. 306; italics my own)

As these proto representations of self and other begin so early in life, it is evident how disrupted attachments, neglect, and other traumatic experiences can have a significant bearing on *expectation* and the way in which reality is perceived. This therefore has important implications for the representation of trauma in phantasies and internal working models: it is often not a single traumatic event which contributes to pathogenic phantasy formation but the repetitious 'micro-depressions' which become early 'schemas' for the repetitive nature of the curse position and the subject's perpetual return to it (Stern, 1994, p. 12). Stern calls these representative forms 'temporal feeling shapes', which are proto-representations embedded within sensory, affective, and temporal experience in the right hemisphere. These are the neurobiological elements of unconscious phantasy and procedural memory which may be prominent factors in terms of generating the uncanny feeling of malediction (Schore, 2009; Stern, 1994, p. 9). The curse then becomes a part of representational experience which is a *weird*, dissociative state of affective homelessness.

Binding the Curse: Uncanny Misfortune

I have set out the contributory historical events for the archaic unconscious in Chapter 1, but here I consider the influence of this archaic unconscious on unconscious phantasy and the curse position.

Hutton's concept of 'uncanny misfortune' is a particularly germane aspect of the archaic unconscious for the curse position (2017). Hutton describes a primal and intergenerational fear of *maleficium*, or supernatural attack.

> There is very little doubt that in every inhabited continent of the world, the majority of recorded human societies have believed in, and feared, an ability by some individuals to cause misfortune and injury to others by non-physical and uncanny ('magical') means.
>
> (Hutton, 2017, p. 10)

This universal fear of *maleficium* relates not only to the concocted fantasies of elite medieval European demonologists of early modern Europe but also to the

Ancient Mesopotamian fear of demons and their malevolent intent (Hutton, 2017, p. 47; Waters, 2019, p. 97). Robin Briggs postulates that this fear of witchcraft – or its equivalent fear of supernatural forces – may be innate to all human beings and passed down intergenerationally:

> A psychic potential we cannot help carrying around within ourselves as part of our long-term inheritance.
>
> (in Hutton, 2017, p. 10)

Given its archaic origins, this primal fear may stem from an unconscious which shares images and affects which are 'archaic' and 'typical' – archetypal (Kalsched, 1996, p. 88). Jung posits a prehistorical deep time where the archetypal system he originally identified may originate:

> Over the whole of this psychic realm there reign certain motifs, certain typical figures which we can follow far back into history, and even into prehistory, and which may therefore legitimately be described as 'archetypes'.
>
> (Jung et al., 2014, p. 179)

An archaic and typical memory system may provide a reasonable explanation for the innate feeling that one has been cursed and the uncanny familiarity which the individual experiences. This archaic memory system may also play an influencing role in the formation of unconscious phantasy, traumatic memories, and the way in which the outside world is perceived. Melanie Klein refers to a 'deeper unconscious' which contains 'terrifying figures' and a savage 'defusing' super-ego formed of the early terrors of psychic disintegration (Klein, 1997, p. 243). Although Klein does not suggest these entities are 'archetypal', her belief that unconscious phantasy is pre-Oedipal leaves room for the possibility of phylogenetic inheritance.

> These extremely dangerous objects give rise, in early infancy, to conflict and anxiety within the ego; but under the stress of acute anxiety they, and other terrifying figures, are split off in a manner different from that by which the super-ego is formed, and are relegated to the deeper layers of the unconscious.
>
> (Klein, 1997, p. 241)

The dissociative or splitting psychic process that Klein describes, where these 'terrifying figures' become split off into a 'deeper' unconscious, evoke the *daimonic* entities described by Kalsched and Jung:

> a diabolical aspect of every psychic function that has broken loose from the hierarchy of the total psyche and now enjoys independence and absolute power.
>
> (Jung, 1953, p. 69)

The 'diabolical aspect' therefore is the shadow side of the *daimon*:

> The Greek words *daimon* and *daimonion* express a determining power which comes upon man from outside, like providence or fate, though the ethical decision is left to man. He must know, however, what he is deciding about and what he is doing. Then, if he obeys he is following not just his own opinion, and if he rejects he is destroying not just his own invention.
>
> (Jung, 1979, p. 27)

The *daimon* is a familiar spirit with independent agency. It is an inner guide which, like intuition, can either be helpful or destructive to the subject. As Jung indicates however, the *daimon* exists outside of the subject's free will and therefore cannot be controlled – as the Faustian myth warns us.

In *The Uncanny*, Freud describes the destructive, '*daemonic*' drive of self-sabotaging behaviour, noting that 'whatever reminds us of this inner "compulsion to repeat" is perceived as uncanny' (1919, p. 238). This archaic, *daimonic* aspect of the unconscious is therefore – given its relation to time and fate – an important driver of unconscious phantasy and the uncanny sense of familiarity in the curse position. We may therefore think of each self-sabotaging act of the curse position which the individual experiences as uncannily familiar as a warning reminder from the familiar spirit/*daimon* which one may choose to either heed or ignore. As Jung importantly notes, the *daimon* is, after all, the one in control of fate and our instincts, and should we choose to ignore its message, we will become – like Macbeth – entirely at the mercy of the forces of fate.

For Donald Kalsched, the *daimon* and its dual nature are central to his theories in the *Inner World of Trauma* (1996). Kalsched describes the way in which the individual develops a 'self-care system' as a result of relational trauma. This *daimonic* archetypal system he describes seeks to protect the individual by mobilising an idealised 'guardian angel' which attempts to shield the subject against the hurt and vulnerability that has become so familiar but, in doing so, becomes 'diabolical and attacks the ego and its vulnerable inner objects' (Kalsched, 1996, p. 45).

The Primary and Secondary Curse

As we have seen, unconscious phantasies and their defences contribute to the looping narratives of the curse position by significantly distorting object relations. I now set out the psychodynamics of the curse position and the subject's attempts to symbolise unconscious phantasy and trauma.

The Primary Curse

The primary curse consists of an unconscious collection of self – object experiences, trauma, and phantasies which attempt to represent (but cannot fully symbolise) experiences of victimisation, alienation, and impingement. The primary curse is also driven by the aforementioned 'temporal feeling shapes' which consist of sensory, affective, and temporal experience in the right hemisphere. Given that these elements have a pivotal role in procedural memory formation, they may also help to explain the traumatic re-enactments of the curse position and the consequent formation of the *affective identity* of a cursed subject. The primary curse may also contain the *daimonic* and uncanny aspects of the 'deeper unconscious'.

The Secondary Curse

The secondary curse is the pre-conscious and conscious experience of the primary curse's 'spell'. Once dominated by the phantasies of the primary curse, the subject *seals the fate* of the position by making a valiant but self-destructive attempt to symbolise them: this then becomes the secondary curse. Unconscious phantasy and trauma also become psychically wrapped up in the pseudo-symbolisation of the secondary curse. The results of this psychodynamic process are represented in the ego as narratives relating to uncanny misfortune: '*Why do these things always happen to me? I must be cursed*', – or its equivalents. The secondary curse therefore becomes a masochistic and omnipotent means of persecutory attacks on the self which mirror or evoke the unconscious phantasies of the primary curse. As a result of the sometimes overwhelming nature of unconscious phantasy and its distorting and sometimes hallucinatory nature, this may create savage superego attacks on the self, high levels of paranoia, or even psychosis. The subject may also project what has now become an overwhelmingly punitive omnipotence into other people or even supernatural entities. In such cases, maleficent misdeeds and intentions may be attributed to others, as in cases of accusations of witchcraft or other forms of 'black magic'.

It is important to note that the secondary curse – as a result of the failure of the ego's attempts to shield itself from the disturbing nature of unconscious phantasy – may also mutate into the dissociative 'fantasying' that Winnicott describes. Due to these dissociative ego defences failing to symbolise unconscious phantasy, the ego is highly vulnerable to the distortions originating in the primary curse. When the ego is dominated by the influence of its more powerful primary developmental antecedent, the individual begins to make 'symbolic equations' which are attempts to symbolise proto-narrative experiences (Segal, 1957). This renders all events and object relations subject to the equative surmises of weirdness, badness, and uncanny misfortune, all tell-tale signs of the secondary curse: '*I've always been weird*', '*I'm an unlucky person*', '*I've always been the black sheep of the family*'.

As will become clear throughout this book, clients who have experienced the relational trauma that leads to the curse position have often become highly attuned to the needs of their caregivers and go on to develop a 'clairvoyant' level of intuition (Ferenczi, 1988, p. 200). Despite the potentially helpful nature of this intuition in terms of personal agency, until the trauma of the curse position is resolved, clients will often continue to ignore their own 'gut instincts' and actively seek out self-sabotaging experiences. Psychotherapy therefore may be an important means of 'lifting the curse' as the therapist sensitively highlights ways in which the client does this in their life and in the transference relationship.

Lifting the Curse: The Witch and the Sorcerer

In Chapter 1, we saw how curse tablets and figurines in the Ancient Greek world were *bound* with curses by sympathetic magic. The early Graeco-Roman procedure of nailing down or manipulating the limbs of 'voodoo dolls' or, later, using written curse tablets represented the misfortune which was hoped would befall their adversaries (Ogden, 2002, p. 245). Importantly for the ancients, the action of cursing could only be conducted by a supernatural entity or a sorcerer. This historical example can provide an analogy, then, with the psychodynamics of the curse position and the way in which the individual attempts to recover lost agency: in unconscious phantasies which are driven by the archaic layers of the unconscious such as that which Hutton identifies, the primary curse is 'believed' to have been placed upon the individual by a supernatural agency such as a sorcerer or witch. Magical practices, therefore, potentially offer traumatised people a means of empowerment and an opportunity to symbolise the primary curse more effectively and integrate traumatic experience. Moreover, as noted in Chapter 2, Frederic Myers – like Donald Kalsched – both see the capacity of the traumatised individual to access a powerful mythopoetic imagination which one may think of as the creative side of the *daimon* (Kalsched, 1996). This *daimonic* magical consciousness can then be harnessed for more harmonious life experiences. However, it should be noted that if the individual remains unconscious of an identification with the mean, manipulative, or aggressive elements of the witch/sorcerer, then the shadow side of the *daimon* continues to dominate object relations and results in traumatic enactments rather than its sublimation.

'Who Is This Who Is Coming'?

M.R. James's 'Oh, Whistle and I'll Come to You, My Lad' is a well-known early twentieth century short story which also draws upon the occult and folklore. I have found this tale useful in terms of illustrating the curse position, particularly in relation to unconscious phantasy and its interaction with the archaic aspects of the unconscious. On a psychological level, 'Oh, Whistle and I'll Come to You, My Lad' dramatises the conflict between the rational defences of the ego and a much more powerful arcane and *daimonic* unconscious.

The story's protagonist, Parkins, is a rather fusty and sceptical academic who is set to go on a combined scholarly and golfing expedition to the east coast of England. An archaeologist colleague asks him to reconnoitre the ruins of an old Templar preceptory. After settling into his accommodation at the Globe Inn, where he has been booked into a large twin room, he plays a round of afternoon golf with his new acquaintance, Colonel Wilson, who is also staying at the Globe. That evening,

Parkins spontaneously decides that he would like to make his own way back to the Inn, perhaps with a view to exploring the Templar site en route.

Among the ruins, Parkins finds an ancient metallic object which he decides to keep. As he walks along the blustery shoreline back to the inn, he perceives a spectral figure who appears to be pursuing him yet which oddly never seems to make up any distance between them. As a result of the bleakness of his seaside walk and the sudden presence of the figure, Parkins begins to feel lonely and craves a companion of his choice rather than the uncanny entity in pursuit. He then thinks back to an 'unenlightened' time in his life when he had read about 'meetings in such places which even now would hardly bear thinking of' and becomes preoccupied by obsessive thoughts of a scene from *The Pilgrim's Progress* concerning a meeting between a Christian and a fiendish entity (p. 63). Parkins then anxiously begins to fantasise of how he might respond if he were to look behind him and the figure were to mutate into a horned and winged demonic entity.

Back at the inn, Parkins cleans the object of its ancient mud, and it reveals itself to be a whistle, upon which there is a Latin inscription on each side: QUIS EST ISTE QUI VENIT and FUR FLA FLE BIS. Parkins manages to translate the former as *Who is this who is coming* (p. 64). To his subsequent detriment Parkins is unable to translate the portentous warning of the latter text, which essentially communicates, *Whoever blows the whistle will live to regret it*. The whistle is ergo protected by a curse. Through either being blissfully unaware of the implications of his actions or hubristically ignoring them, Parkins then blows the whistle and, as he does so, immediately sinks into a hypnotic reverie:

> It was a sound, too, that seemed to have the power (which many scents possess) of forming pictures in the brain. He saw quite clearly for a moment a vision of a wide, dark expanse at night, with a fresh wind blowing, and in the midst a lonely figure – how employed, he could not tell.
>
> (p. 65)

Parkins's reverie is then followed by a gust of wind which is so intense that it blows the candles out in his room (p. 66). That night, as he vainly tries to sleep, Parkins is persistently preoccupied by persistent inner visions of a figure running in terror from an assailant, 'in pale, flickering draperies, ill-defined', though this time the assailant appears to be making up the ground between them (p. 67).

The next morning, one of the hotel staff comments to Parkins that the second bed in his room also seems to have been slept in. Parkins is consequently disturbed, as he can see no suitable rational explanation for this. He departs for another round of golf with Colonel Wilson. Clearly indicating his own belief in folkloric wisdom and the forces of sympathetic magic, the Colonel comments on the heavy winds of the previous night and how these may have been summoned by the act of whistling. Parkins, ever consciously the sceptic, quickly dismisses this as foolhardy superstition. Nonetheless, when Parkins discloses his whistling activities of the previous night, the Colonel tells him that he would be wary of keeping the object, indicating that, given its origins, the possibility might be subject to 'Papist' sorcery (p. 70). As the two men make their way back to the inn, they bump into a boy who is running away in terror from the very inn where they are staying. After interviewing him, it transpires that he has been terrorised by a non-human entity which was waving at him from Parkins's bedroom window. When the two men arrive at the Globe and enter Parkins's room, it appears that the other bed in his room has once again been disturbed. Parkins shows the Colonel the whistle, but the Colonel can make nothing of the inscription in the poor light. Nonetheless the Colonel says that were the whistle in his possession, he would return it to the sea as soon as possible, though he already understands that Parkins will not heed his counsel. As he retires that night, Parkins is subsequently attacked by the phantom occupant of the other bed, who lunges for him with a face of 'an intensely horrible, face of crumpled linen' (p. 76). As the phantom attacks Parkins, the Colonel dramatically enters the room. As he does so, Parkins faints, and the phantom is now just a 'tumbled heap of bed clothes' (ibid.). However, as the author notes, it is not clear whether the bed-linen phantom could have done physical harm to Parkins other than the psychological harm it causes him.

Discussion

The threatening entities of the story are *weird* in the sense that they are '*ill defined*' shapeshifting humanoids which do not belong (James, 1987, p. 67; italics my own). The whistle is an instrument of sympathetic magic which summons the demonic entity and the accompanying maleficent wind (Frazer, 1994). According to Frazer, this form of sympathetic magic is a form of sorcery: '*Do this in order that so and so may happen*' (Frazer, 1994, p. 32).

Importantly, it is not only the whistling action which summons the evil entity but Parkins's initial careless uncovering of it at the Templar site. This suggests the existence of an ancient sorcery which the curious should not meddle with, such as that of the myth of the curse of Tutankhamun (Luckhurst, 2014). As we recall from Jung's statement on the *daimonic* connection to fate, Parkins's assailant may therefore be an apparition of his own *doppelgänger*. It is not clear over which shoulder Parkins looks, but the way in which the phantom shapeshifts from a rather ineffectual phantom – perhaps an initial warning vision – into a much more threatening *fiendish* entity suggest an indirect allusion to Ancient Egyptian lore with regard to *sinistration* and the taboo of looking back.[3]

The Egyptians believed that to look back over the left shoulder and see one's *Ka* (one's soul or spirit – in Greek terms, *daimon*) signified an ill omen (Bateson, 1923, p. 242). To see one's *doppelgänger* is also more widely believed in folklore to be an omen of one's imminent death. In these terms, the *Ka* is not only a manifestation of a *daimonic doppelgänger* but also a mythological antecedent to the *sinister*, which etymologically relates to the left side and its association with bad luck and evil intent. Looking back is also a taboo relating to the curse of Orpheus.

Parkins's inner visions are driven by his own previous fascination with a dark supernatural which he has now dissociated, resulting in the emergence of frightening entities such as those which feature in the meeting between Christian and 'fiend' – a reference to the demon Apollyon in Bunyan's *The Pilgrim's Progress*. The destructive mythological figure of Apollyon is a return of a repressed entity from the deeper levels of Parkins's unconscious, unleashed as a result of his disrespectful actions. His inability to translate the all-important Latin taboo inscription may also be considered part of the destiny which has been written for him but which he is barred from knowing; his fate is lost in translation. The Colonel's warning is also a taboo: Parkins must not whistle, as according to seafaring lore, whistling 'raises the wind' which is associated with witchcraft, jinne spirits, and danger (Hole, 1967; O'Neill et al., 2015). Although the scene when Parkins is attacked by crumpled bed linen is perhaps rather comical in some respects, it does also point to the traumatic terror of confusion between inside and outside, absence and presence.

'Oh, Whistle and I'll Come to You, My Lad' is an entertaining fable which warns against disavowal of one's archaic unconscious and the wisdom of its omens. By ignoring archetypal wisdom and the advice of those around us, we can become captured by the potency of the destructive *daimon* and lose the protection of its benign counterpart. Blowing the whistle then comes to represent one of the most powerful yet underestimated acts of sorcery – when a curse is unconsciously placed upon the self and becomes a self-fulfilling prophecy.

Clinical Illustration: *The Fourth Stone*

Mr. G., a man in his early forties, sought therapy as he was suffering from what he described as anxiety, depression, and overwhelming guilt over his father's death. Although Mr. G. was clearly a gifted photographer and had been complimented by many people over the years – including a small but not insubstantial following on social media – he continued to work in what he described as 'boring office jobs which pay the bills'. Mr. G. said that he had been given opportunities to 'follow his dreams' as a photographer but could never muster the courage to go fully freelance. He had also been offered some funding for a photography project but turned it down. When I asked him why he had done this, Mr. G. said that he had always had the profound feeling that success was something for other people, and failure was what he had come to know best. Anyway, he was too old now, he said. I remember feeling an intense sadness at this moment, combined with a bubbling up of irritation. There was something quite aggressive about Mr. G.'s dismissal of his ambitions and somehow nihilistic expectations of what therapy could achieve. It felt like he was denigrating the work that we had agreed to do together.

Mr. G. was very aware of how he contributed to his own 'failure'. He told me that he wasted a lot of his free time watching TV or 'doom scrolling' on his phone instead of doing what he 'really' wanted to do: taking photographs. He said it annoyed him when people would say that photography was his 'hobby', as he felt that was patronising. The denigrating nature of this reference to the outside world struck me once again. He earnestly added that he thought that people were right to call it a hobby, as, although it felt like something much more than a hobby to him, unless he gave up his day job, that's all it would ever be.

Mr. G. had never sustained a long-term relationship, though he really hoped he could now meet someone he could 'settle down with'. He said that he had always found relationships difficult, as he would choose partners 'with problems' and whom he enjoyed 'helping out' at the beginning but then would find the pressure on him overwhelming and end the relationship.

Mr. G.'s father had been unfaithful to his mother multiple times, which everyone in the family knew, but this was never spoken about openly. He was a vain, narcissistic man who worked in financial services. His moods were highly unpredictable and would quickly switch from manic episodes of elation to fits of rage, often when his brittle ego felt slighted. Mr. G. told me that he had always been afraid of his father.

Mr. G.'s father favoured his older brother, who had followed in his father's career footsteps and now ran his own hedge fund. Although Mr. G. said that he felt his mother loved and cared for him, she was often preoccupied by her own anxieties about her disintegrating marriage. Mr. G. took it upon himself to try to make his mother feel better, and although this was temporarily successful, it would never be long before things reverted to the way they were.

Mr. G. had a keen interest in *Dungeons and Dragons* as a teenager, and his 'tough guy' brother and his friends would sometimes berate him for this. He had also been bullied at school and been the recipient of similar taunts there, particularly by boys he described as 'macho'. Notwithstanding its relationship to bullying, Mr. G. said that *Dungeons and Dragons* and reading fantasy and horror fiction at this time brought him great comfort, and, along with the camaraderie this brought with others with similar interests, this had been the beginning of an exploration of a metaphysical, ineffable reality that he had always felt a connection with since he was a child.

When Mr. G. was in his early thirties, he had a dream which would shatter his world dramatically:

I'm standing on an industrial wasteland, something like a brownfield site. There is old farming machinery everywhere and it's really scary, kind of like the Texas Chainsaw Massacre. *It's foreboding. In the middle of the scene there are three standing stones. I feel captivated by them as they seem so ancient and incongruous with the rest of the scene, but it also somehow seems right. I become aware of a strong beam of sunlight illuminating the stones and I feel a sense of relief, as if I'm escaping something, or being offered a chance of some kind. I don't know what exactly. But then I notice that to the left of the scene there is a small area of the site that has a strange twilight, as if it's in a separate time zone somehow. Slowly I can see a dark mass emerging from the twilight and I can see that this is a fourth stone. It is gnarly and full of malevolent intent, as if it wants to cause me great harm. Somehow I knew that this meant my father's death was imminent and I woke up terrified, in a cold sweat.*

The following week Mr. G.'s father had a fatal heart attack. Mr. G. had not spoken to his father for several months and subsequently fell into a deep depression, overcome by the feeling that he had been personally responsible for his father's demise: he had come to equate his uncanny ability to foresee his father's death with the magical power to actually cause it. The guilt began to 'eat him up' and he couldn't shake the idea that the hatred that he had always felt for his father had now finally killed him off.

Mr. G. said that he did not leave the house for two months after his father's death. The GP signed him off work, and he spent most of his time eating takeaways, drinking cheap lager, and chain-smoking roll-ups. His financial situation had forced him back to work, yet he had still done no photography. Mr. G. told me that his father's death confirmed what he had always suspected – that he had been doomed since he was born, and his mere existence was a curse on everyone else.

I felt a twinge of that annoyance again that had now become quite familiar. Although Mr. G. acknowledged his hatred for his father and accompanying death wish, he otherwise spoke as if he were incapable of having aggressive feelings towards other people. He would put his own misfortune down to the fact that, in his words, he was 'a despicable human being'.

We continued to work through the dream. Mr. G. said that the setting of the dream felt to him like the atmosphere of the family house growing up and that old farming machinery made him think about how much he hated the world and how it had become mechanised and controlled by technology. He said that this was 'a farm that had been disbanded millennia ago – that's my family – always left behind by time'. He looked full of sorrow when he said this, and there were tears in his eyes. He paused and wiped the tears away, and as he spoke, his voice tremored as he tried to suppress his crying. 'I'm sorry', he said.

I asked him why he was sorry.
'I don't know really, I guess I don't want to make you feel worse'.
'Worse how?' I asked.
'Well, I guess I don't wanna be a burden on anyone', he replied. 'I always felt like that with my mum – like I was afraid of making her feel worse if I shared my problems. In the end I just presumed that I was the problem I 'spose'.

The way that Mr. G. said 'I 'spose' struck an affective chord of nostalgia somewhere deep inside of me. Somehow, I was reminded of when he told me that he was 'too old'. 'I 'spose' was a such a simple phrase, but the way he abbreviated it sounded anachronistic for someone of his age, as if he had perhaps copied his parents' idiosyncratic way of saying 'I 'spose' as a child, and it had stuck with him. Sometimes when he said it, I imagined a little boy wanting to please his mother, using her phrase to show her he was a grown-up – that he was *old enough*.

After sitting with this for several moments, I realised that despite the tender feelings that I felt for Mr. G., I was conscious of once again colluding with his defence against rage and disappointment:

> 'If you never felt that your feelings really mattered to anyone, did that also include your negative feelings?' I asked.
>
> 'Yes, I guess so'.
>
> 'Could this be why you hate conflict so much?'
>
> 'Maybe'.
>
> 'It's just that I'm really wondering about that *Texas Chainsaw* bit of the dream', I added.
>
> Mr. G. laughed. 'Ha, yeah, good point', he said. 'Well, I 'spose that's the atmosphere that we often had at home. Growing up in that house I knew I always had to be on my guard . . . to second-guess how my dad would behave – it felt *menacing* you know . . . but in a way I think because I was so scared of him, I seem to see a lot of horrible creatures in my dreams'. [Mr. G. had shared his dreams quite often and they did indeed often contain a wide range of eldritch beings.]
>
> 'What about your dad? How do you think your terror of him has affected your relationship to anger?' I asked.
>
> He paused for a moment and said, 'I've always felt that anger was the enemy, so I've always made sure I keep it inside . . . It terrifies me to think of it 'cos there is a part of me that feels like a monster. But I don't want to feel like that anymore. I know that I need to find a way to tell people when I don't want to do things, or I don't like things without feeling like a monster'.
>
> 'Is there anything you'd like to tell me?' I asked. Mr. G. looked slightly perplexed.
>
> 'Like what?'
>
> 'About what you don't like, or don't want to do in therapy'.
>
> 'OK, well yeah, I guess I could say something. . . . Sometimes these sessions seem like a waste of time and I don't want to come. It's taking such a long time, and that annoys me sometimes. I feel like it shouldn't take so long', he said.
>
> I knew from previous sessions that he tended to use the word 'annoyed' euphemistically, so I asked him about it. I wanted to help him move away from the self-censorship he had learned in his family.
>
> 'Would you say you were angry about that?' I asked.
>
> He laughed nervously and then thought for a few moments. 'Yeah, I 'spose it does'. There was anguish in his eyes, as if he feared a retaliation. When he could see that this was not forthcoming, he looked relieved.
>
> 'Yes, therapy does take time, and I can appreciate that makes you frustrated and angry sometimes', I replied.

There was a long pause, perhaps as long as a couple of minutes: as if it were a telepathically agreed time-out for reverie.

I broke the silence by asking Mr. G. what he made of the stones.

'Which ones?' he asked, now half smiling.

'Whichever, I guess', I replied.

'OK – Well you know in Japan number four is super unlucky. So, I've always been a bit scared of it and have tried to avoid it if I can – OCD I know! [He laughs nervously again.] So I think that's why it has that horrible menacing feeling in the dream. Though it's weird because I've actually realised that my dad's birthday is on the 4th as well – probably why I want to avoid it'. He laughed nervously again. I found this funny inwardly, but there was a biting undertow which I found myself resisting against.

He paused for some moments. 'I'm sorry, I'm feeling a bit choked up again now. [He paused again, and the tears returned to his eyes.] It's really annoying, but I actually miss my dad now, or maybe I miss the dad I wanted but didn't have. I just wish that I'd had a dad who was normal and loved me like other people's dads do. [He thought for a few moments before continuing.] You know, now I'm actually thinking that the other three stones are me, my mum, and my brother. That dream also makes me realise that I wanted dad out of our lives so badly for so many years, so I 'spose that explains that feeling of chance, opportunity . . . the feeling that if we could only be without him, everything would be OK . . . so that the sun would finally shine on us three. The problem is there's actually no way to get rid of that fourth stone and that horrible twilight – he will always darken our door! That twilight never ends – it's part of me. Like that fourth stone is always there as a reminder of dad. I 'spose I'd always wanted the special powers to kill him off, just to *erase* him without anyone knowing, turn him to stone, like the trolls in *The Hobbit*'. He laughed again; I then felt the deep sadness that perhaps Mr. G. did not wish to feel at that moment.

As therapy continued, we returned to the 'fourth stone' dream every so often, and Mr. G. could now begin to grieve his wished-for father. He had also reconsidered his perspective on the fourth stone and understood that it could also represent himself and the way that he always felt like an outcast in his family. He also began to rebuild a relationship with his brother, who had long battled cocaine addiction, and found a way to form stronger emotional boundaries with his mother, whom he had also encouraged to attend therapy, which she was now considering. He still hadn't found anyone to begin a committed relationship with but felt more confident that he was in a better place to do so. He also continued to slowly take ownership of his own anger. Mr. G. was now much more inclined to let me know if there was something that I had said or done that he disagreed with, rather than making denigrating comments and disowning them. He still tried to avoid direct conflict if he could, but the thoughts and phantasies around it had lost some of their potency. There were also less frequent reports of monstrous creatures and psychopathic assassins in his dreams. He said that he missed those dreams in a way, as he thought they would be useful creatively, but not the feeling that went with them.

Mr. G. now realised that he could never escape from his real family and its real past. He said that the three stones not only represented his wished-for family but also an 'old and wise' part of him which reminded him of his passion for photography and creativity in general: he also linked this with a non-idealised feeling of chance and opportunity that the three stones transmitted. After attending weekly therapy for three years, Mr. G. informed me that he had had his first photography exhibition, which had gone 'pretty well'. On the back of this, he had also been commissioned and received funding to work on a local project and could therefore afford to go part-time at work.

Discussion

As a result of the symbolic equations of the primary curse, Mr. G. had developed a hallucinatory, Oedipal gratification that killing off his father would free him of his own demons. He wished for a transcendent Neverland where he would live with the remaining members of his family – symbolised by the three stones. Therapy therefore offered him a means of gentle 'disillusionment' from this phantasy rather than the violent impingements and abandonments that he had experienced at home (Winnicott, 1982, p. 17).

It is important to emphasise that Mr. G.'s wish to kill his father was not purely based on an Oedipal drama but on a very real traumatising terror of his father and emotional abandonment by his mother. There is instead a convergence of the Oedipal wish of a traumatised self that confronts a mythical unconscious, all of which bear down on unconscious phantasy and the primary curse. Mr. G.'s wish to turn his father to stone illustrates this meeting of psychic forces – 'like the trolls in *The Hobbit*' and the synchronicity between the 'unlucky' number four and his father's birthday. The 'twilight' of the fourth stone represents Mr. G.'s guilty wish: the fourth stone therefore came to symbolise the 'weird', *unheimlich* internal object: that which does not belong but can never be magically erased. Jung pertinently notes how the *quaternio* comes to represents the unifying opposites between the chthonic/spiritual and good/evil (1978 p. 63). Therefore, despite Mr. G.'s omnipotent desire to magically remove his father from the family – the evil entity in the *quaternio* – the remaining three family members can only ever aspire to an illusory wholeness.

The fourth stone and the *Texas Chainsaw* atmosphere of the dream represent a threatening prehistory from where the dream entities and Mr. G.'s fear of his own murderous rage emerge. Mr. G.'s dread of the 'unlucky' number four also links to his dread of a foreboding prehistorical time which holds the power to curse his fate. The number four therefore becomes 'unlucky', as his *Texas Chainsaw* aggression towards his father does not match his cursed identity. 'Unlucky' number four also represents his feelings of cursed misfortune in the family as he identifies with the 'scapegoat archetype' (Perera, 1986):

Individuals identified with the scapegoat archetype feel themselves to be the carriers of shamefully evil behaviors and attitudes that disrupt relationships – that discomfort the parental figure.

(Perera, 1986, p. 15)

The identification with the scapegoat archetype therefore becomes part of the secondary curse, part of Mr. G.'s 'despicable' identity.

There is a notable convergence in this case between different forms of nostalgia and its etymological associations with home, pain, and homesickness. There is an archaic, transcendent nostalgia transmitted by the prehistoric standing stones in the dream which intersect with Mr. G.'s sorrow for his family, which had – like the stones – been 'disbanded' and 'marginalised by time'. Mr. G. had become an 'old soul' before his time: like his family, the standing stones, and the trolls, it was too late for him to change. Yet my countertransference to the way in which he said 'I 'spose' indicated something quite different – a nostalgic desire for 'holding' and mirroring (Winnicott, 1982).

It would be easy to write off the precognitive nature of the dream as wish fulfilment and Mr. G.'s father's subsequent death as coincidence rather than meaningful synchronicity. Yet the *wyrd* and prophetic nature of the dream and his father's subsequent actual death led to what Kripal calls

traumatic transcendence – that is a visionary warping of space and time affected by the gravity of intense human suffering.

(2020, p. 35)

Mr. G. had also developed a high level of emotional intelligence and intuition, and there were certainly times in the sessions when I felt we were psychically connected in a way which felt close to telepathy, as if we were in *daimonic* dialogue. The dream therefore became an important 'transitional object' which enabled Mr. G. to experience his feelings of vulnerability and 'burden'-like dependency in the transference and to begin to reflect upon them as opposed to acting them out by denigrating his therapy (Winnicott, 1982). This mutual reverie meant that Mr. G. could begin to harness his intuition as part of his alpha function rather than perceiving it as a 'beta' threat from the primary curse (Bion, 1984). I was also able to draw upon the *Texas Chainsaw* atmosphere of the dream to help Mr. G. begin to assimilate and mentalise his rage rather than only see himself as a victim of his father's narcissistic abuse and to find a means of expressing his anger in the transference without retaliation.

Concluding Comments

This chapter has described the contributing psychic elements which combine to form unconscious phantasies and the importance of pre-narrative psychic phenomena in the formation of the curse position. I have described the way in which trauma and the *daimonic* unconscious can also have a significant bearing on unconscious phantasy and its role in attempts to symbolise traumatic experiences of failures of absence and presence. Through the topographic model of the curse position, we have seen the way in which traumatic experiences result in failures of symbolisation and self-sabotaging repetition compulsions. Given the sense of uncanny misfortune that is so central to the curse position and the uneasy unconscious relationship between *heimlich* and *unheimlich* internal objects, the archetypal and *familiar* nature of intuition is therefore potentially perceived as a threat to the subject – the uncanny shadow side of the *daimon*. Therapy therefore offers an arena where the working alliance can be a means of helping clients to reconnect with the intuitive self. Importantly, in this respect, this intuitive familiar becomes part of alpha function, rather than relegated to 'instinct' alone; dissociated as part of *beta* elements; or used as an omnipotent, auxiliary self (Bion, 1984). Familiars also provide a means of contact with the ancient world through their association with shamanism, witchcraft, and fairy lore (Wilby, 2005).[4]

The ego has to be shaken to revitalize the familiar. Therefore poets and painters move where its veils are most transparent – in the realms of love, death and vision. They follow the path of ancient gods, whose outer forms were in harmony with the forces they enshrined. They love ruins because of the intense nostalgia they induce for the return of infinite space to where it had been so rigidly limited.

(Grant, 2021, p. 39)

Acknowledgements

My thanks to Will Kearney for his inspiring comments on the transcendent nature of nostalgia.

Notes

1 These definitions are elaborated upon further in Chapter 4.
2 Fisher does not appear to say, however, whether with regard to the weird and the eerie that there is an equal reluctance to acknowledge the inside.
3 Taboo: 'Do not do this, lest so and so should happen' (Frazer, 1994, p. 32).
4 There are further encounters with familiar spirits in Chapter 6.

References

Bateson, H. (1923). Looking over the left shoulder. *Folklore*, 34(3): 241–242.
Beebe, B. and Lachmann, F. M. (1988). The contribution of mother-infant mutual influence to the origins of self- and object representations. *Psychoanalytic Psychology*, 5(4): 305–337.
Bion, W. (1984). *Learning from Experience*. London: Maresfield Library.
Bohleber, W., Jiménez, J. P., Scarfone, D., Varvin, S. and Zysman, S. (2015). Unconscious phantasy and its conceptualizations: An attempt at conceptual integration. *The International Journal of Psychoanalysis*, 96: 705–730.
Breuer, J. and Freud, S. (2004). *Studies in Hysteria*. London: Penguin.
Bunyan J. and Owens W. R. (2008). *The Pilgrim's Progress*. Oxford University Press.

Davies, J. M. and Frawley, M. G. (1992). Dissociative processes and transference-counter-transference paradigms in the psychoanalytically oriented treatment of adult survivors of childhood sexual abuse. *Psychoanalytic Dialogues,* 2(1): 5–36.

Erreich, A. (2015). Unconscious fantasy as a special class of mental representation: A contribution to a model of mind. *Journal of the American Psychoanalytic Association,* 63(2): 247–270.

Ferenczi, S. (1988). Confusion of tongues between adults and the child – The language of tenderness and of passion. *Contemporary Psychoanalysis,* 24: 196–206.

Fisher, M. (2014). *Ghosts of My Life: Writings on Depression, Hauntology and Lost Futures.* Winchester: Zero Books.

Fisher, M. (2016). *The Weird and the Eerie.* London: Repeater Books.

Frazer, J. and Fraser, R. (1994). *The Golden Bough.* Oxford: Oxford University Press.

Freud, S. (1919). The 'Uncanny'. In Freud, A., Strachey, A., Strachey, J, and Tyson A. (Eds.), *The Standard Edition of the Complete Psychological Works of Sigmund Freud, Volume XVII (1917–1919): An Infantile Neurosis and Other Works.* London: Hogarth Press and the Institute of Psychoanalysis pp. 217–256.

Freud, S. (2004) *Hysterical Phantasies and their Relation to Bisexuality.* In Breuer, J. and Freud, S. (2004). *Studies in Hysteria.* London: Penguin.

Grant, S. (2021). Mage and Image. In K. Grant and S. Grant (eds), *The Carfax Monographs.* Somerset: Fulgur Press.

Grotstein, J. (2008). The overarching role of unconscious phantasy. *Psychoanalytic Inquiry,* 28(2): 190–205.

Hewitt, M. A. (2020). *Legacies of the Occult: Psychoanalysis, Religion, and Unconscious Communication.* Sheffield: Equinox.

Hole, C. (1967). Superstitions and Beliefs of the Sea. *Folklore,* 78(3): 184–189.

Hutton, R. (2017). *The Witch.* New Haven: Yale University Press.

Isaacs, S. (1948). The nature and function of phantasy. *International Journal of Psycho-Analysis,* 29: 73–97.

James, M. R. (1987). *Casting the Runes and Other Ghost Stories.* Oxford: Oxford University Press.

Jung, C. G. L., Hull, R. F. C., Read, H., Adler, G. and Fordham, M. (1953). The Collected Works of C. G. Jung. Volume 12 Psychology and Alchemy. London: Routledge & Kegan Paul.

Jung, C. G. L. (1978). *Aion: Researches into the Phenomenology of the Self.* Princeton: Princeton University Press.

Jung, C. G. L., Adler, G. and Hull, R. F. C. (2014). *Collected Works of C.G. Jung, Volume 16 Practice of Psychotherapy.* Princeton: Princeton University Press.Jung, C. G. L., Hull, R. F. C., Read, H., Adler, G. and Fordham, M. (1953). *The Collected Works of C. G. Jung. Volume 12 Psychology and Alchemy.* London: Routledge & Kegan Paul.

Kalsched, D. (1996). *The Inner World of Trauma: Archetypal Defenses of the Personal Spirit.* London: Routledge.

Klein, M. (1946) Notes on Some Schizoid Mechanisms. In *Envy and Gratitude and Other Works* 1946–1963 (3rd edn). London: Vintage.

Klein, M. (1997). On the Development of Mental Functioning. In *Envy and Gratitude and Other Works 1946–1963* (3rd edn). London: Vintage.

Kripal, J. (2020). *The Flip: Who You Really Are and Why it Matters.* London: Penguin.

Kristeva, J. (1982). *Powers of Horror: An Essay on Abjection.* New York: Columbia University Press.

Laplanche, J. and Pontalis, J. B. (1973). *The Language of Psycho-analysis*. London: The Hogarth Press and the Institute of Psycho-Analysis.

Luckhurst, R. (2014). *The Mummy's Curse: The True History of a Dark Fantasy*. Oxford: Oxford University Press.

O'Neill, S., Gryseels, C., Dierickx, S., Mwesigwa, J., Okebe, J., d'Alessandro, U. and Peeters Grietens, K. (2015). Foul wind, spirits and witchcraft: Illness conceptions and health-seeking behaviour for Malaria in the Gambia. *Malaria Journal*, 14(167).

Ogden, D. (2002). *Magic, Witchcraft, and Ghosts in the Greek and Roman Worlds*. Oxford: Oxford University Press.

Ogden, T. H. (1984). Instinct, phantasy, and psychological deep structure: A reinterpretation of aspects of the work of Melanie Klein. *Contemporary Psychoanalysis*, 20: 500–525.

Perera, S. (1986). *The Scapegoat Complex: Toward a Mythology of Shadow and Guilt*. Toronto: Inner City Books.

Schore, A. N. (2009). Right-Brain Affect Regulation: An Essential Mechanism Of Development, Trauma, Dissociation, and Psychotherapy. In D. Fosha, D. J. Siegel and M. F. Solomon (eds), *The Healing Power of Emotion: Affective Neuroscience, Development & Clinical Practice*. New York: W. W. Norton & Company, pp. 112–144.

Segal, H. (1957). Notes on symbol formation. *The International Journal of Psychoanalysis*, 38: 391–397.

Segal, H. (1994). Phantasy and reality. *International Journal of Psycho-Analysis*, 75: 395–401.

Spillius, E. B. (2001). Freud and Klein on the concept of phantasy. *The International Journal of Psychoanalysis*, 82(2): 361–373.

Stern, D. (1992). The 'pre-narrative': An alternative view of 'unconscious phantasy' in infancy. *Bul. Anna Freud Centre*, 15: 291–318.

Stern, D. N. (1994). One way to build a clinically relevant baby. *Infant Mental Health Journal*, 15(1): 9–25.

Waters, T. (2019). *Cursed Britain: A History of Witchcraft and Black Magic in Modern Times*. London: Yale University Press.

Weiss, H. (2021). The conceptualization of trauma in psychoanalysis: An introduction. *The International Journal of Psychoanalysis*, 102(4): 755–764.

Wilby, E. (2005). *Cunning Folk and Familiar Spirits: Shamanistic Visionary Tradition in Early Modern British Witchcraft and Magic*. Brighton: Sussex Academic Press.

Winnicott, D. (1965). The maturational processes and the facilitating environment: Studies in the theory of emotional development. *The International Psycho-Analytical Library*, 64: 1–276 (London: The Hogarth Press and the Institute of Psycho-Analysis).

Winnicott, D. (1982). *Playing and Reality*. London: Routledge.

Winnicott, D. W. (2018). *Psycho-Analytic Explorations*. London: Routledge.

Chapter 4

The Curse Position (2)

The Uncanny

Introduction

Given the significant influence of Freud's essay *The Uncanny* on the formation of the concept of the curse position, selected elements from that essay have already been introduced in Chapter 3. Here, I wish to elaborate on Freud's paper and E.T.A. Hoffman's 'The Sandman'. Each provides an important insight into the relationship between the uncanny and its hermeneutic connection to the repetitively destructive relationships to self and others. Both of these texts also provide early and foundational insights into the concept of the *doppelgänger* and its relation to the superego, the archaic unconscious, and the compulsion to repeat. Building on Freud's concepts, I have added my own clinical perspectives on relational trauma and the uncanny. I also argue that the uncanny provides a portal which grants us access to magical consciousness and psychic faculties which can prove helpful in times of difficulty, and I provide a personal example of this.

Trauma & The Uncanny: What Comes to Light

Early on in his essay, Freud defines the uncanny as

> that class of the frightening which leads back to what is known of old and long familiar.
>
> (1919, p. 220)

He adds further texture by also citing Schelling's definition of the phenomenon:

> the name for everything that ought to have remained secret and hidden but has come to light.
>
> (1919, p. 224)

These two definitions connect the time and space elements of the uncanny and indicate the existence of archaic elements which will always eventually make themselves known. In his essay, Freud builds further on these definitions through

DOI: 10.4324/9781003168027-5

a conscientious analysis of an etymology of the uncanny and demonstrates that although the *unheimlich* (unhomely) may indicate something fearful or eerie, it does not necessarily follow that the *heimlich* (homely) equates to the 'cosy' side of the familiar. Much trauma takes place in the setting of the *heimlich* (the home), which then becomes a source of shame and guilt that the family seeks to conceal through the defences which are most familiar to them: the '*heimlich* places'. The following definition that Freud selects for the *heimlich* is therefore hauntingly apposite (1919, p. 223):

> To do something heimlich, i.e. behind someone's back; to steal away heimlich; heimlich meetings and appointments; to look on with heimlich pleasure at someone's discomfiture; to sigh or weep heimlich; to behave heimlich, as though there was something to conceal; heimlich love-affair, love, sin; heimlich places (which good manners oblige us to conceal).

Heimlich places perhaps exist then to conceal what cannot be spoken about. However, a closer look reveals only an opaque veneer through which traces of deception can be perceived. This is germane for the trauma at the kernel of the curse position, as the former has a complicated relationship with the truth – 'what comes to light' and how it can be spoken about in psychotherapy. As Freud asserts, the *heimlich/unheimlich* are by no means antonyms but themselves curious chameleo-doubles which have the capacity to take on one other's signifying properties (1919, p. 224). The uncanny resists simple definition, or perhaps even any definition at all.

'The Sandman'

'The Sandman' is an unsettling, phantasmagorical tale with an ahistorical feel written by E.T.A. Hoffmann, widely considered to be one of the early pioneers of weird fiction (Hoffmann, 2012). I state that 'The Sandman' is unsettling as it can be read as an unfolding of a psychotic breakdown as a result of the failure of the reliance on primitive, narcissistic defences. Indeed, Hoffmann shows a profound understanding of psychopathology without ever needing to use clinical terminology. One can see, then, why this story from this perspective alone would have appealed to Freud, but it also enables him to explore and develop his own ideas, particularly around the uncanny aspects of the Sandman as a myth, mechanical objects, *doppelgängers*, and the eyes and their relationship to the castration complex. Although Freud includes a summary of 'The Sandman' in *The Uncanny*, I have written a version below as an accompaniment/alternative.

'The Sandman': A Summary

'The Sandman' tells the story of Nathaniel and the events which take place in his childhood and as a young man relating to the figure of the Sandman. 'The Sandman' is based on a German folkloric figure who either benignly sprinkles sand on children's eyes (as Nathaniel's mother reassures him) or removes their eyes to feed his own children (as Nathaniel's Nanny warns him). Nathaniel initially believes the Sandman to be a demonic lawyer called Coppelius.

Coppelius visits Nathaniel's father early in the story, where each appear to be involved in an alchemical experiment. When Nathaniel interrupts them in their occult endeavours, Coppelius threatens to take Nathaniel's eyes out. Nathaniel is saved from this fate by his father's protestations, yet that does not stop Coppelius from unscrewing Nathaniel's hands and feet and putting them back together again as if he were a toy. Nathaniel then awakes, and it is not made clear to the reader – particularly given its grim absurdity – whether this horrific act actually took place or was a product of Nathaniel's florid oneiric phantasy. This bizarre passage – with particular regard to this unscrewing of Nathaniel's limbs – serves as an initial portentous signifier of the *human as automaton* which recurs in the story and which Freud also discusses in *The Uncanny*. Coppelius then devastatingly murders Nathaniel's father, which Nathaniel believes is part of a Faustian pact that his father had unwisely signed up for. Although the reader is to assume the murder *really has* taken place – as will become clearer as the story unfolds – the line between phantasy and reality is thin in 'The Sandman', and Hoffmann therefore provides the reader with a window into Nathaniel's deeply troubled and confused psyche.

After the murder of his father, Nathaniel's state of mind now rapidly deteriorates, and he receives a letter from his sweetheart Clara which is full of tenderness and concern for his now profoundly disturbed state of mind, lovingly cautioning him against confusing persecutory phantasy with external reality.

As Clara becomes increasingly concerned about Nathaniel's out-of-control paranoia, she begs him to see reality. Indeed, Clara comes across as a compassionate rationalist, and Hoffmann makes it clear she has no time for airy mysticism. Nevertheless, as is clear to clinicians working with psychosis, attempting to disprove the existence of supernatural phenomena through 'logical disputation' to those who suffer with annihilation anxiety of a psychotic kind only leads to further states of fear and alienation (McWilliams, 2011, p. 18). Despite her best intentions, Nathaniel's narcissism is only therefore further wounded by what he unjustly perceives as Clara's pedestrian rationality. Despite the resilience of Nathaniel's solipsistic persecution complex, Clara is occasionally able to get through to him, yet only fleetingly, at one point managing to persuade him that Coppelius the lawyer and Coppola the salesman are not really the same person.

Nathaniel begins to attend the lectures of a physics professor called Spalanzani, who bears some resemblance to the 18th century occultist Cagliostro, a further allusion, perhaps, to alchemy. Nathaniel then becomes fascinated by Spalanzani's daughter Olympia, though he notices that there is something unusual about her. Nathaniel returns home and attempts to put his paranoid phantasies into poetry, depicting Coppelius as the evil sorcerer who has cursed his and Clara's love and transformed it into a death's head out of which Clara's eyes uncannily stare. In his petulant grandiosity, Nathaniel expects Clara to be instantly swept away by his poetic genius. Clara is, of course, not remotely impressed and refuses to gratify his narcissistic demands. In retaliation, Nathaniel refers to Clara as a mechanical doll – the second reference to the automaton in the story.

Nathaniel returns to his studies only to find that his apartment has burned down, though his friends have kindly saved his possessions for him. Nathaniel then quickly finds new lodgings, yet only to once again be haunted by the doubling of Coppola/Coppelius – this time in the guise of Coppola the barometer salesman. It initially appears to Nathaniel that Coppola wishes to sell him eyes but then realises that Coppola means an instrument to aid sight. Given the aforementioned uncanny uncertainty around what things actually *are*, it is difficult to be sure, but this proposed instrument appears to be something along the lines of binoculars –which Nathaniel then decides to buy. Nathaniel subsequently uses a specular instrument to spy on Olympia in Spalanzani's apartment. Once again, the reader is now shown a disturbing window into Nathaniel's psyche. Through Hoffmann's ingeniously oneiric mutating symbols, at this point in the story, we are in touch with a bewildering sense of existential uncertainty: is this instrument a magnifying glass, a pair of binoculars, some spectacles, or a mirror? These symbiotic signifiers suggest that whatever Nathaniel sees is a product of his narcissistic imagination and is, therefore, the font of much of his delusion.

Nathaniel is next invited to a party hosted by Spalanzani where Olympia is to make her public debut and perform a piano recital. After Nathaniel watches Olympia's recital in an enraptured state, they dance together, at which point he declares his love for her despite her clearly robotic characteristics.

It is now the turn of Nathaniel's university friend, Siegmund, to become tarnished by Nathaniel for being the unfeeling rationalist, as he now expresses concern for Nathaniel's love for what everyone else can see is obviously a doll. Nathaniel blithely ploughs on regardless, deciding that he will marry Olympia anyway, but his amorous bliss is interrupted by a violent wrestle for custody of Olympia between Coppola/Coppelius and Spalanzani, where one party holds her by the shoulders and the other by the feet. Coppola eventually escapes with Olympia, and the way in which he carries her finally makes it clear to Nathaniel that she is an automaton. In the midst of Coppola's escape, Nathaniel notices Olympia's disembodied eyes are staring up at him from the floor, which Spalanzani then picks up and throws at him. Nathaniel then flies into a psychotic rage and attacks the professor, attempting to strangle him before bystanders intervene to save the professor from certain murder. Nathaniel returns home and now expresses gratitude to his friend Siegmund for not abandoning him.

Now returning home again, Nathaniel seems to begin to recover, back in the care of Clara, his mother, and friends. One day, Clara and Nathaniel decide to climb the town hall tower. As they look out from the summit, Clara notices an uncanny bush-like object that appears to be approaching them. Nathaniel then takes out the eye/looking glass that Coppola had sold him from his pocket and this time looks at Clara through the lens. Nathaniel is immediately possessed by another murderous episode, and Clara now appears to him as if she were a wooden doll. He then attempts to throw her from the tower, though she is saved by her brother Lothar. At the end of the story, Coppelius reappears (now back in the guise of the lawyer) at the foot of the tower, predicting that Nathaniel will come down of his own volition. At the sight of Coppelius, Nathaniel falls to his death.

Commentary

The *doppelgänger* is an important manifestation of the uncanny, as it is a phantasised realisation of its recurrent, shapeshifting aspect. Indeed, there is much doubling, shapeshifting, and recurring throughout 'The Sandman': things appear to be the same, but they are uncannily different, even if it is not clear why. The Sandman figure may be a benign metaphor for aiding children's sleep or a threatening and violent psychopath who steals their eyes. Coppelius and Coppola are also chameleo-doubles, and Nathaniel's inability to split them indicates that these might be manifestations of unconscious phantasy of narcissistic trauma. Freud writes,

> They are a harking-back to particular phases in the evolution of the self-regarding feeling, a regression to a time when the ego was not yet sharply differentiated from the external world and from other persons. I believe that these factors are partly responsible for the impression of the uncanny, although it is not easy to isolate and determine exactly their share of it.
>
> (Freud, 1919, p. 236)

Freud also posits that, as the Sandman provokes a narcissistic disturbance, Nathaniel's fear of intimacy becomes a fear of castration, so in this way Coppelius becomes the evil, split-off aspect of his father that is intolerable. Surely, though, if this is a fear of castration, then rather than a literal terror of genital mutilation, it is a fear of psycho-somatic disintegration, which Winnicott calls 'falling forever' (1974, p. 103), and is symbolised by the screwing off of Nathaniel's limbs.[1] Nathaniel's phantasy is thus an example of what McWilliams classifies as a psychotic defence stemming from terror:

> Probably the most important thing to understand about people with psychotic illnesses or psychotic-level psychologies is that they are terrified. It is no accident that many drugs that are helpful for schizophrenic conditions are major antianxiety agents; the person with a vulnerability to psychotic disorganization lacks a basic sense of security in the world and is ready to believe that annihilation is imminent.
>
> (McWilliams, 2011, p. 87)

I would nevertheless agree with Freud's interpretation that Nathaniel's love is narcissistic: Nathaniel's love is only a schizoid phantasy that his 'love' objects – Clara and Olympia – may remain only as automatons, without any of the complications of contending with an actual living and breathing subject.

> We may with justice call love of this kind narcissistic, and we can understand why someone who has fallen victim to it should relinquish the real, external object of his love.
>
> (Freud, 1919, p. 232)

Freud therefore interprets this in terms of the castration complex as the explanation for his phantasy, and this perhaps works if the castration anxiety is used as a broad metaphor to indicate a fear of intimacy: it is Nathaniel's fear of the bad object – represented by the Sandman – which leaves him unable to have a relationship with a human being.

> The psychological truth of the situation in which the young man, fixated upon his father by his castration complex, becomes incapable of loving a woman, is amply proved by numerous analyses of patients whose story, though less fantastic, is hardly less tragic than that of the student Nathaniel.
>
> (ibid.)

At another point in *The Uncanny*, Freud argues – quite categorically – that children do not fear 'living dolls' (p. 233). On this point, I would beg to differ: the idea of a living doll coming to life in daylight may seem benign, but when the gloaming of the evening arrives, it may take on threatening features. In this scenario, it is the terror of things *not being as they 'should'* which is uncanny. In his short story 'The White People', Arthur Machen defines this as a particular form of 'sin':

> What would your feelings be, seriously, if your cat or your dog began to talk to you, and to dispute with you in human accents? You would be overwhelmed with horror. I am sure of it. And if the roses in your garden sang a weird song, you would go mad. And suppose the stones in the road began to swell and grow before your eyes, and if the pebble that you noticed at night had shot out stony blossoms in the morning?
>
> (Machen, 2011, p. 113)

Machen's 'sin' may be read as an illustration of the Winnicottian paradigm of trauma unpredictably impinging upon the predictable (Winnicott, 2018, p. 198). Nathaniel's 'love' for Olympia may be considered as an allegory of a traumatic enactment of impingement on infant reality: by falling in love with the impinging object (the automaton), he can master and control it: an obsessive, portentous phantasy has completely taken over Nathaniel's psyche.

With the curse position there is no control, no 'real' free will, for free will is itself illusory, and the cursed subject is therefore bound to the mercy of the threatening and wordless affects of the primary curse; the superego guilt-based defence of the secondary curse only adds voices of judgement and shame to the mix. Nathaniel's inability to control fate and its relationship to the reminding omen is laid down early in the story with the depiction of himself as a doll with detachable limbs, which then recurs in Olympia and in Clara. In this way, fate itself becomes symbolised by the mechanical doll that Nathaniel deludes himself that he can control by means of his psychotic vision of love, yet he cannot escape the 'cold and prosaic' reality of death. Indeed, for Freud. the *doppelgänger* – like the automaton – is not only a portentous double, but also a manifestation of superego (Freud, 1919, p. 235): in narcissistic or 'primitive' reality, the double is 'an insurance against the destruction of the ego', and superego is therefore its successive double, though superego 'reverses' the 'assurance of immortality' into 'the uncanny harbinger of death' (1919, p. 235). In defences such as paranoia, there is thus a consequent perceived threat to the self which creates the uncanny sense of being watched. One form of omnipotence is in this way exchanged for another; as feelings of immortality are no longer available and the reality of death becomes apparent, paranoia and 'knowing one's enemies' become a shoring up against it (ibid.). The watchful agency recurs in 'The Sandman' in the form of the double and also in the various ocular manifestations we encounter along the way, the latter also perhaps a reference to the evil eye, which we will encounter again in Chapter 9.

With these references to this 'watchful agency', Freud implicitly alludes to other significant meta-psychological papers, such as the 'watchful' conscience found in *Mourning and Melancholia* (1917) and *The Ego and Id* (1923) and the 'ego-ideal' of *On Narcissism* (1914). Freud also recounts his own experience of this agency. While travelling by train, he realises to his 'dismay' that the 'elderly gentleman' he has seen in the carriage was in fact only his own reflection, whose appearance he 'thoroughly disliked', which one might *speculate* is a shattering of Freud's ego-ideal by his superego (1919, p. 248).

For Freud, then, the uncanny double is a reminder of the archaic unconscious: a period in history 'long since surmounted'; indeed, it would be terrifying if one were plunged back into it without warning and, indeed, why severe states of regression can be highly destabilising in therapy (1919, p. 236). Freud postulates that the uncanny is, therefore, in part a 'throwback' to the animistic and symbiotic world where the boundaries between self and other are not well defined, though he cannot be certain of the degree to which this creates the uncanny effect (ibid.). He therefore acknowledges that there will always be cracks in 'progress' through which the uncanny can enter though still maintains that it evolves from an inferior and regressive form of mental functioning. This also applies to the uncanny effect of seeing meaningful patterns or synchronicities as superstitious phantasies that can be traced back to infancy (1919, p. 238). As we have seen in the previous chapter, at the heart of Freud's argument there is a positivist assumption that the magical, animist consciousness of 'primitive man' is something that 'we in the West' have largely 'surmounted', and the uncanny is its residue: a return of the repressed. I would certainly agree that the repression of the archaic unconsciousness explains the appearance of uncanny derivatives in dreams, synchronicities, parapraxes, and traumas, yet the devaluing of this consciousness to a rudimentary stage of development in Freud's argument certainly requires revision. Therefore, instead of the uncanny representing a return of the repressed derivatives of a 'primitive' or narcissistic stage of development, they become a reminder of humanity's violent dissociation from nature and the natural world, along with the artificiality of the barrier which has been constructed between ourselves and the (super)natural world. The uncanny in this sense is by no means a regression but a signifier of 'intrusive familiars' from the archaic unconscious which offer phenomenological experiences of magical consciousness such as the uncanny, synchronicity, divination, and telepathy: *these entities have become threatening as they have become repressed* (Staley, 2011). The uncanny therefore becomes a means of accessing magical consciousness. In this form of consciousness, I would include Jung's synchronicity and the numinous (1969), Wilson's superconscious (2015), Myers's mythopoetic experience and 'the subliminal self' (see Taves, 2003), and Fisher's *The Weird and the Eerie* (2016).

The Compulsion to Repeat

Another key concept of Freud's *The Uncanny* which has become useful clinically and in the development of the curse position is the 'compulsion to repeat' (ibid.). Freud observes that, as this is such a powerful compulsion, it may 'overrule' the pleasure principle and is linked to the 'daemonic' aspects of mind present at early stages of psychic development and in neurotic patients, the latter of whom exhibit omnipotent and superstitious phantasies such as seeing repetitive patterns which would otherwise be attributed to chance (ibid.). Although Freud's thesis is here based on his economic model of mental functioning and, in this respect, differs from the largely object relations and trauma-based aetiology of the curse position, he nonetheless captures the 'daemonic character' of the compulsion that applies to each case (ibid.). Moreover, writing in *Beyond the Pleasure Principle* one year later, Freud describes another aspect of the repetition compulsion, which Laplanche and Pontalis call 'fate neurosis', which also contains this essential 'daemonic' element which is powerfully evocative of the curse position and the sense of being *victimised* by uncanny misfortune (1973).

> The impression they give is of being pursued by a malignant fate or possessed by some 'daemonic' power.
>
> (Freud, 2001, p. 21)

In this 'passive' population that Freud highlights, unlike neurotics, bad things seem to simply happen in this particular neurosis without their involvement; hence, this becomes a uniquely *daimonic* form of repetition compulsion (Freud et al., 2001, p. 22). The presence of the *daimon* – and it is a malignant *daimon* in this case – emphasises the lack of agency the subject has and also how baffling cases of the compulsion to repeat can be for not only clients but also their therapists. The uncanny and *daimonic* aspect of the repetition compulsion that Freud pinpoints therefore provides an important clinical perspective on the curse position and its relationship to developmental trauma.

Much trauma takes place within the environment of the home – the *heimlich* – and relational or developmental trauma is caused by shocks to subjectivity which take place there and is most damaging in the years between birth and the age of four (Gaensbauer and Jordan, 2009). As a result of the relational trauma that takes place in this early period of life, the individual searches for strategies of control that will instil the certainty that was absent at the time of the trauma and which then become a particular kind of tyranny of rigidity which generates what Janet calls 'fixed ideas' (Van der Hart and Horst, 1989). The uncanny's affective echoes therefore stem from this early point of disintegration where the *unheimlich* (unfamiliar) attempts to fuse with the *heimlich* (familiar) and is experienced as a devastating attack on infant subjectivity, as it is the familiar which is the bad object to which they return (Fairbairn, 1943; Van der Kolk, 1989).

Developmental trauma manifests later in life in a 'fear of breakdown' – of what has not yet happened yet which has, paradoxically, already taken place (Winnicott, 1974). This dissonant psychic storm creates a fissure over which a psychic scar forms: the primary curse. Each time the trauma that formed the scar is activated through traumatic memories[2] and unconscious phantasies, there is no signified present: the scar only serves as a reminder of a cursed past and an omen of a repeating future. This interaction between unconscious phantasy and trauma is what makes working clinically with the repetition compulsion so complex, and attempts to disentangle the two are likely to frustrate clients and therapists, particularly as the wishes associated with unconscious phantasy often result in the defences of repression and dissociation (Bohleber, 2007).

The Keystone

While I was writing this book, I experienced a series of events which are pertinent to this conjunction between the uncanny and magical consciousness and which revolved around my office and the coronavirus pandemic. This was a time of collective uncertainty and anxiety, in lockdown. Many colleagues had already decided to resign their leases in their offices and to work from home. However, in my case, although I could see that it made sense to work remotely from home, it hadn't been long since I had taken up the lease, and I had become attached to the space and hoped that I might find a way to return to in-person work before long. This inner conundrum would last for several months.

One December evening during the first winter lockdown of 2020, while taking a break between clients, I was sitting reading in preparation for an upcoming chapter of this book. I was positioned opposite a bookcase, over which I could see the top of the office window. I could also see that it was now dark and raining heavily outside.

At some point I heard a huge *thwack* and immediately afterwards saw a large black, amorphous object fall through the ceiling in the area between the bookcase and the window. Although I couldn't see what it was, the object seemed to have landed on the floor with a tremendous *bang*. In a state of shock, I thought that the ceiling had subsided and whatever had landed on the floor had come through the hole. After a few more moments, I looked up at the ceiling, and it became quickly clear that it was as before. Feeling somewhat puzzled, yet equally fascinated, I then wondered what could have caused the sound and inwardly hypothesised that, as double-decker buses frequently passed the office, one of these might have simply created an audio-visual illusion: the shadowy object had simply been a reflection of a bus through the frosted glass window. Nonetheless, this didn't seem to account for the fact that *I had clearly seen an object falling through the ceiling* and then heard the subsequent crashing sound. At that point, I thought it therefore feasible that a book had fallen from the shelf which caused the sound, so I went around the side of the bookcase to have a look. I was stunned to see that there were indeed *two* books on the floor – Mark Fisher's *The Weird and the Eerie* and *Capitalist Realism*. Aside from the fact that these were both books by the same author, they are relatively short, and weigh very little; only a weighty hardback dropped from a great height could have made such a sonic impact. As I stood in a mildly befuddled stupor, I strongly sensed that this had been a supernatural practical joke – a visitation from the archaic unconscious by a mischievous trickster.

In the subsequent months, I remained unsure of the best course of action to take, until the following events took place that would help me reach a final decision as to whether I should stay or go.

At lunchtime one beautiful spring day, I went to let myself out of the office, and my key broke clean in half inside the lock. I managed to tease the remaining half out, though, as I now only had a broken key, I couldn't open the door until my wife arrived to let me out from the other side using a spare copy. I was struck by the singularly affective nature of this event, which I intuitively felt to signify an important message regarding my continuing dilemma, though at this stage, I was still not in a position to decipher what it communicated.

The following day, I went to the local newsagents, and the man in front of me went to get some change out of his pocket. Somehow in the process of doing so, he managed to break his house key clean in half. I was amazed to see that the two halves he held up to the shopkeeper in dismay looked identical to my own and also that his key had broken in the same place as mine.

That evening, while recounting the above events to a friend on the telephone, I suddenly felt struck by a strong compulsion to tell him about a particular passage in Robert Aickman's 'The Cicerones' (1990) as somehow I felt that this also related to my dilemma. Bizarrely, I didn't know which passage it was I needed to tell him about, but I *did* know that it was relevant to our conversation – I felt very much at this stage that my unconscious was in control, and I just needed to follow it.

The very brief passage describes a man who has become trapped inside a crypt in a Belgian cathedral at the end of a sequence of disturbing interactions with the cicerones (the guides), and the image he perceives on a keystone above a door in the crypt appears to represent his ultimate fate: a demonic kidnapping of his soul.

I was taken aback by the way in which, through the process of reading Aickman's tale, it had been this particular passage which had chosen to lodge itself in my unconscious as if it were a spell – without my awareness – and then remained there as a cipher until it revealed its meaning at this moment of speaking to my friend. Indeed, as I read the passage out to my friend, I then felt quite clear that my unconscious had 'known' something which I had consciously hitherto not – that this passage would mean something important to me. I could not say exactly why, yet I felt quite sure that this short paragraph was in itself 'the keystone': that which held everything together and meant something significant to me. Although I couldn't identify a specific 'demon' that was relevant to my conundrum, the symbol was nonetheless chilling, and it somehow represented the 'crypt' of indecision that I had become trapped in for some time. The demon which appears at the end of the story also evoked a potent trickster mischief similar to that which I had encountered in the office. This unruly and archaic entity heralded the entry of an uncanny and turbulent indecision but also came to represent its resolution. *The Cicerones* was ergo not only a tale of the uncanny, but a magical *grimoire* whose spell guided me towards the all-important decision that had evaded me for so many months: it was now definitely time to leave my office.

Commentary

I have chosen to set out the events above as they illustrate the conjunction between the uncanny and magical consciousness, and despite their often disturbing or numinous nature, if we can pay attention to their signs and symbols, they can become important resources. The sequence of events I experienced also illustrate the important connection between traumatic events and numinous experiences that Kripal calls 'traumatic transcendence':

> a visionary warping of space and time effected by the gravity of human suffering.
> (Kripal, 2020, p. 35)

The intense collective trauma of the pandemic was perhaps, therefore, the genesis of the strange and sometimes inexplicable events which took place and my subjective reaction to them, which felt profoundly meaningful to me.

Although my initial conundrum as to whether I should have left my office or not may, on the face of it, have appeared rather pedestrian as an illustrative example of 'traumatic transcendence', I believe the stasis and anxiety I experienced related to a much deeper collective trauma in society at the time. This trauma then became a psychic tear through which uncanny elements which 'ought to have remained secret and hidden' had now, as a result of the pandemic, 'come to light' (Freud, 1919, p. 224). This sense of 'coming to light' particularly applied to the first experience in my office that took place in December 2020. Everything that happened that strange evening could easily be interpreted rationally, yet on an intuitive and affective level, I somehow felt that I *knew* that this had been a very brief but intense lifting of the veil of time and space reality, and despite its frightening and rather Lovecraftian numinosity, I felt very privileged to have experienced it. I was also quite shaken by the sense that this had somehow been a communication from an *unheimlich* reality that existed outside of the *heimlich* and evoked the phenomenological 'sin' which Machen describes. Though I could not say what the communication meant, I deeply felt that it was connected with the devastating events that were taking place in the world. Indeed, Lacan states that what cannot come to light in the symbolic realm will appear in the real (Lacan and Fink, 2006, p. 324). This very much applied to the pandemic – particularly in the early stages, there was much that could not be thought about, let alone symbolised.

What applies to all of the events that I have described is that there was a perceived link between my inner reality and that which took place in the outside world (Kripal, 2020, p. 147). Jung calls this 'synchronicity' or 'meaningful coincidence' (Jung, 1969). These links between the inner and outer world feel profoundly important, yet as Jung affirms, they cannot be explained intellectually:

> This is necessarily the case when space and time lose their meaning or have become relative, for under those circumstances a causality which presupposes space and time for its continuance can no longer be said to exist and becomes altogether unthinkable.
>
> (Jung 1969, p. 654)

With incidences of the uncanny, synchronicity, and traumatic transcendence, the familiar laws of space and time become redundant. In such cases there is often a gripping feeling of awe or even terror which cannot be conveyed. Kripal's concept of 'traumatic transcendence' may provide a helpful link here between the concepts of magical thinking and consciousness: the trauma of the scenario which I found myself in during the pandemic perhaps may be interpreted as an omnipotent state of mind, yet it was also this magical thinking which led me towards the meaningful coincidences that would become helpful to me. By shedding light upon the recurring symbol of the key, my unconscious became a cicerone which guided me away from a split 'either/or' state of mind towards a 'depressive position' where I was finally able to make the decision to leave my office and begin to mourn what had taken place and what might have been had it not (Klein, 1997).

Concluding Comments

The ideas which are manifest in *The Uncanny* are pivotal to the curse position, particularly with regard to the way in which each relates to the double, the superego and the *daimonic* nature of repetition compulsion. Perhaps as a result of *The Uncanny's* somewhat meandering nature, it almost presents itself as work of fiction rather than concerning issues of such clinical importance, though its great strength is perhaps that it manages to do both. Through the story of 'The Sandman', we have seen the way in which the narcissistic defences can lead people onto 'a dangerously destructive path', and it therefore reminds us as clinicians that reality testing is not sufficient to work with such grandiose and paranoid-schizoid states of mind. I have also considered how the role of the archaic unconscious and developmental trauma interact with one another and described through a personal example the way in which the uncanny can become the gateway to magical consciousness where the *daimon* takes on a guiding, rather than purely destructive, role.

Notes

1 See Freud's footnote 1 in *The Uncanny*.
2 Under the umbrella of memories, I include affects, memories, flashbacks, dreams/night-mares, and bodily sensations.

References

Aickman, R. (1990). The Cicerones. In *The Unsettled Dust*. London: Faber & Faber.

Bohleber, W. (2007). Remembrance, trauma and collective memory: The battle for memory in psychoanalysis. *International Journal of Psychoanalysis*, 88(2): 329–352.

Fairbairn, R. (1943 [1952]). The Repression and the Return of Bad Objects (with Special Reference to the 'War Neuroses'). In W. R. Fairbairn (ed), *Psychoanalytic Studies of the Personality*. London: Routledge and Kegan Paul.

Fisher, M. (2016). *The Weird and the Eerie*. London: Repeater Books.

Freud, S. (1914). On Narcissism. In Freud, A., Strachey, A., Strachey, J, and Tyson A. (Eds.), *The Standard Edition of the Complete Psychological Works of Sigmund Freud, Volume XIV (1914–1916): On the History of the Psycho-Analytic Movement, Papers on Metapsychology and Other Works*. London: Hogarth Press and the Institute of Psychoanalysis. pp. 67–102.

Freud, S. (1917). Mourning and Melancholia. In Freud, A., Strachey, A., Strachey, J, and Tyson A. (Eds.), *The Standard Edition of the Complete Psychological Works of Sigmund Freud* (Vol. XIV). London: The Hogarth Press and the Institute of Psychoanalysis.

Freud, S. (1919). The Uncanny. Freud, A., Strachey, A., Strachey, J, and Tyson A. (Eds.), In *The Standard Edition of the Complete Psychological Works of Sigmund Freud, Volume XVII (1917–1919): An Infantile Neurosis and Other Works*. Hogarth Press and the Institute of Psychoanalysis pp. 217–256.

Freud, S. (1923). The Ego and the Id. In J. Strachey (ed), *The Standard Edition of the Complete Psychological Works of Sigmund Freud, Volume XIX (1923–1925): The Ego and the Id and Other Works*. London: The Hogarth Press and the Institute of Psychoanalysis, pp. 19–28.

Freud, S., Strachey, J., Freud, A., Strachey, A. and Tyson, A. (2001). *The Standard Edition of the complete Psychological Works of Sigmund Freud: Early Psycho-Analytic Publications. Volume 18 (1920–1922) beyond the Pleasure Principle Group Psychology and Other Works*. London: Vintage.

Gaensbauer, T. J. and Jordan, L. (2009). Psychoanalytic perspectives on early trauma: Interviews with thirty analysts who treated an adult victim of a circumscribed trauma in early childhood. *Journal of the American Psychoanalytic Association,* 57(4): 947–977.

Hoffmann, E. T. A. (2012). *The Sandman*. London: Penguin.

Jung, C. G. (1969). *The Structure and Dynamics of the Psyche* (2nd edn). Princeton: Princeton University Press.

Klein, M. (1997). *Envy and Gratitude and Other Works 1946–1963* (3rd edn). London: Vintage.

Kripal, J. (2020). *The Flip: Who You Really are and Why it Matters*. London: Penguin.

Lacan, J. and Fink, B. (2006). *Ecrits: The First Complete Edition in English*. London & New York: W.W. Norton.

Laplanche, J. and Pontalis, J. B. (1973). *The Language of Psycho-analysis*. London: The Hogarth Press and the Institute of Psycho-Analysis.

Machen, A. (2011). *The White People and Other Weird Stories*. Oxford: Oxford University Press.

McWilliams, N. (2011). *Psychoanalytic Diagnosis Understanding Personality Structure in the Clinical Process*. New York: Guilford Press.

Staley, M. (2011). The Resurgence of Cosmic Identity. In A. O. Spare, *The Book of Pleasure (Self Love): The Psychology of Ecstasy*. London: Jerusalem Press.

Taves, A. (2003). Religious experience and the divisible self: William James (and Frederic Myers) as theorist(s) of religion. *Journal of the American Academy of Religion*, 71(2): 303–326.

Van der Hart, O. and Horst, R. (1989). The dissociation theory of Pierre Janet. *Journal of Traumatic Stress*, 2: 397–412.

Van der Kolk, B. A. (1989). The compulsion to repeat the trauma: Re-enactment, revictimization, and masochism. *Psychiatric Clinics of North America,* 12(2): 389–411.

Wilson, C. (2015). *The Occult*. London: Watkins Books.

Winnicott, D. W. (1974). Fear of breakdown. *International Review of Psycho-Analysis,* 1(1–2): 103–107.

Winnicott, D. W. (2018). *Psycho-Analytic Explorations*. London: Routledge.

Chapter 5

The Ancestral Curse

This chapter explores various ways that the curse is passed down through the generations through secrets which are sequestered in the layers of the deep unconscious through Holocaust trauma, post-slavery syndrome, and economic inequality. Indeed, the memories, fixed ideas, phantasies, and dissociated affects are perhaps the most obvious aspects of trauma that one may think are inherited and become the source of repetition compulsion, yet one may easily overlook that the defences are also 'incorporated' (Abraham and Torok, 1994). These defences are often dissociative in nature, and the research of Liotti (2004) points to a link between intergenerational trauma, disorganised attachment, and dissociation. The chapter ends with a study of post-slavery syndrome and its relationship to intergenerational trauma and transference dynamics.

Ghosts 1: The Phantom: Sacred Scars

Despite the significance of the curse of Oedipus and unconscious repetition for Freud, notwithstanding the fact that they are certainly implicated in much of his work, there is no explicit reference to intergenerational transmission of trauma in his writing. Despite this absence, Fonagy points to Freud's 'radical' insight on intergenerational trauma in *Totem and Taboo*:

> We may safely assume that no generation is able to conceal any of its more important mental processes from its successor.
>
> (Freud, quoted in Fonagy, 1999)

This quote once again evokes the concealment of the '*heimlich* places' of the family discussed in the previous chapter and the way in which families struggle to metabolise and symbolise trauma, particularly when it is the result of atrocities such as genocide or slavery (Freud, 1919, p. 223). Kestenberg describes the 'transposition' of intergenerational trauma which results in second-generation survivors reliving their parents' trauma (Kestenberg, quoted in Fonagy, 1999, p. 93).

> These are children of individuals onto whom trauma was transposed, who created murdered internal objects on the basis of their interactions with survivors,

DOI: 10.4324/9781003168027-6

who were brought up in a 'world beyond metaphor' but who themselves had no direct experience of trauma.

(Fonagy, 1999, p. 94)

For Auerhahn and Laub, who carried out extensive research on Holocaust survivors, each generation become 'secret bearers' (in Prager, 2016, p. 18). In lieu of a parent's capacity to contain unbearable anxiety, the child instead becomes the container of the parent's trauma (Kogan, in Prager, 2016). Separation and individuation (the child's aspiration to fulfil their own desires) are thus experienced as a betrayal of the secret and a re-enactment of the original trauma (Prager, 2016).

The Encrypted Unconscious

Abraham and Torok describe a traumatic 'phantom' which haunts successive generations (Abraham eand Torok,1994). They postulate that the 'phantom' is no more than 'an invention of the living', though 'what haunts' are not the dead but the gaps left within us by the secrets of others (Abraham and Torok, 1994, p. 171). These 'invented' gaps then leave an ontological quandary: *how are we to fill them, particularly if we do not even know that they are there*? The phantom lies deep in the subject's unconscious and therefore presents an unseen obstacle for psychotherapy:

> The special difficulty of these analyses lies in the patient's horror at violating a parent's or a family's guarded secret, even though the secret's text and content are inscribed within the patient's own unconscious. The horror of transgression, in the strict sense of the term, is compounded by the risk of undermining the fictitious yet necessary integrity of the parental figure in question.
>
> (Abraham and Torok, 1994, p. 174)

This 'fictitious integrity' therefore feeds into the 'moral defence' of the parent where threatened removal of bad objects presents a violent trauma to the client (Fairbairn, 1943). Attempts to 'remove' the bad objects through therapeutic action potentially place the therapist in the seat of the split-off aggressor parent in the transference as the client protects her soul's DNA. The phantom is therefore created by the 'gap' that is internalised: it is what is *not* said by the parents and the resulting phantasies that become lodged in the unconscious of the next generation; I would therefore infer that this is internalisation from nonverbal interactions and gestures; the phantom is an inheritance of what is so markedly not said but what is implied. The gap is what cannot be spoken of in order to preserve the guilt and the shame of the ancestors, which have become sacred scars in the mind of each generation. Abraham and Torok therefore write that this is an *incorporated* guilt and shame (undigested phantasies transmitted by parent to child) rather than the *introjected*, metabolised version of the events which had occurred (Abraham and Torok, 1994). The phantom thus is the product of 'catastrophe' or 'narcissistic injury' that becomes a 'foreign body' which is encrypted into the unconscious and makes itself known in uncanny ways in psychotherapy (ibid.). It passes through the body of each generation as *memories without memory* that become locked in a 'crypt' of the self which resists symbolisation (Abraham and Torok., 1994; Schwab, 2010):

> the phantom which returns to haunt bears witness to the existence of the dead buried within the other.
>
> (p. 175)

Ghosts 2. *Ghosts in the Nursery:* Crimes of the Imagination?

These traumas and the associated guilt and shame form bonds between the generations, linked by phantasmic threads, poignantly illustrated in *The Ghosts in the Nursery*, which compassionately documents clinical work with parents and their children who have been traumatised through successive generations by inequality, poverty, and abuse (Fraiberg et al., 1975). As Fraiberg and her colleagues affirm, there are 'ghosts' in every nursery:

> while no one has issued an invitation, the ghosts take up residence and conduct the rehearsal of the tragedy from a tattered script.
>
> (Fraiberg et al., 1975, p. 388)

The authors state that adverse life events by themselves do not serve to predict that their relationship with their children will be adversely affected but rather *the defences they have developed as a result*. The researchers notice two main defences: identification with the aggressor[1] and isolation of affect. The research subjects often therefore react with hostility towards their children or speak of brutalising experiences in a dissociated, matter-of-fact fashion.

The paper also illustrates a particularly toxic form of unconscious phantasy which Fraiberg et al. call 'crimes of the imagination' (1975, p. 393). With inherited trauma, there is a 'sense of tormenting sin' as one's conscience becomes the perpetrator of violent masochistic crimes against the self, yet the aggressor with which one unknowingly identifies is that of the parents or ancestors (Fraiberg et al., 1975). Fraiberg and her colleagues highlight a tendency among the subjects to remember what happened in instances of trauma, though it is not the memory which becomes the phantom/ghost but its associated affect, which is uncannily absent. Although the authors of the article attribute this defence to repression, I would argue that this would now be considered as a common dissociative response to trauma, where the affects 'take on a life of their own' (Van der Kolk, 2015, p. 86).

The later research of Fonagy and colleagues confirms Fraiberg's hypothesis that the more intractable traumatic hauntings are correlated with parents who tend to use more primitive and dissociative defences. This leads to defensively aggressive and controlling reactions in the infant which are associated with disorganised attachment

(Fonagy, 1999). Moreover, research has highlighted a causative link between mothers who were recorded to have unresolved trauma in adult attachment interviews and children who were diagnosed with a disorganised attachment (Fonagy et al., 1993, Liotti, 2004). Mary Main illustrates how the disorganised attached child that is

> preprogramed to turn to the parent in moments of alarm – is caught between contradictory impulses to approach and avoid. It is an untenable position from which the child's dependency on the parent affords no escape.
>
> (Wallin, 2007, p.22)

This is an ontologically crippling paradox which the infant faces as the parent in whom she seeks security is also the one she is either afraid of or who appears to be afraid (ibid.). Liotti elucidates parallels between disorganised children and their dissociated parents, indicated by the latter's Adult Attachment Interview (AAI) ratings. This also points to the way in which children in the 'Strange Situation' research test one moment show affection towards their caregivers and then suddenly switch to hypnotic or aggressive behaviour, thereby providing plausible evidence for the transmission of intergenerational trauma:

> Since disorganized attachment in children is strongly linked to unresolved AAI ratings in their parents, these observations hint at the possibility of an intergenerational transmission of dissociative mental states that is related to unresolved memories of past parental traumas.
>
> (Liotti, 2004, p. 474)

Fonagy describes the 'bizarre' behaviour of children with disorganised attachment who disturbingly come to physically act out their uncanny ego disturbances:

> when reuniting with their caregiver following a brief period of separation – behaviours such as head-banging, freezing, hitting, hiding, or collapsing.
>
> (Fonagy, 1999, p. 95)

For the infant with an unpredictable caregiver and an insecure subjectivity, these dissociative defences may quickly become the best possible line of defence in order to

> eliminate from consciousness that which interferes with the reestablishment of order and predictability in needed relationships. However detrimental it may be for the traumatized person's perception of reality, dissociation is often crucial to the reestablishment of a sense of certainty about psychological survival.
>
> (Brothers, 2013, p. 7)

The splitting of dissociation is another manifestation of the double: Janet referred to its narrowing of consciousness as *dédoublement* (Van der Hart and Horst, 1989,).

As Brothers postulates, (2013), dissociation is a shoring up against unpredictability, as are its associated defences of a narrowed field of consciousness and 'fixed ideas' (Van der Hart and Horst, 1989,). In today's language of trauma, we see fixed ideas in the flashbacks, night terrors, and panic attacks of PTSD (Van der Hart and Horst, 1989; Van der Kolk, 2015) For Van der Kolk, 'dissociation is the essence of trauma' (2015, p. 6). The dissociative response is driven by limbic, sensory phenomena that operate independently from one another – as presented by patients in *The Ghosts in the Nursery*. However, given the limbic sources of dissociated material often found in PTSD, clinicians such as Van der Kolk advise against the purely abreactive psychoanalytic approaches taken by Fraiberg et al., which, he believes, are inadequate for treatment of the limbic system and may even increase reliance on dissociative defences. He therefore recommends a multifaceted body-based approach and therapies which enable the subject to reintegrate dissociated material and to gently widen their window of tolerance (2015, p. 86).

The Alien Self

As we have seen from the infant research of Chapter 3 on implicit relational knowing and pre-narrative envelopes, subjectivity is formed of a complex network of experience, which includes proto-symbolic memories which enable the infant to begin to make basic predictions and have expectations of external reality, from which unconscious phantasies are formed.

An infant therefore begins to 'look for' herself in the mirrored reactions of caregivers, and the reflections she sees *are* her subjectivity (Fonagy, 1999, p. 103). When parents become dissociated or angered at infant distress, the infant then makes psychic room for an 'alien-self', as her expectations subside in her need to preserve attachment security at whatever cost to her subjectivity, the costly price of which she is, of course, tragically not aware of. This means that the infant fails to see herself as an 'intentional being' in the intersubjective mirror, which then potentially becomes the beginning of her own deficits in mentalisation and later reliance on dissociation (Fonagy, 1999, p. 103). In lieu of the caregiver's recognition of the infant's intentionality, a new phantom subjectivity is internalised based on the parent's aggression, fear, or dissociation, which is 'alien to self-representational structure' (Fonagy, 1999, p. 104). The child's 'true self' therefore becomes concealed within the *heimlich* places of the mind, or the crypt of the deep unconscious. In *The Picture of Dorian Gray*, we may consider the ugly, alien self which Dorian so chillingly locks away in the attic represents the 'alien self' which the infant has no choice but to internalise and 'adopt'.

Clinical Illustration

Parents may desire a better childhood for their own children than they experienced. This desire can, however, itself be a curse, as they may consequently overcompensate. Ms. D., a woman in her late fifties, had a mother who had been emotionally distant, and Ms. D. felt she had never been able to approach her mother about her feelings. She described her father as interfering and controlling 'like a dictator'. Now her own children tell her that she 'micromanages' them, and although they know she is emotionally available, they experience this as an impingement upon their autonomy. It had become a repetition compulsion: each time she wanted to show love and affection for her children, she felt they would withdraw from her.

Ms. D. felt very stuck in therapy for a long time and asked me for 'tips' on how she could help her children through directive advice. She also asked me several times whether I had children myself and was frustrated when I did not answer her question directly. When I asked her why it was important for her to know, she told me that she was afraid I might not understand her.

I said that I could see why she was concerned, as, if told her that I did not have children, she might feel that I couldn't relate to her experience as a parent, but, if I told her that I did, then I would become 'an expert' – like her father – who could manage Ms. D.'s life for her yet wouldn't leave her much space to think for herself. I added that I wondered whether she might experience my lack of a clear answer as a rejection – that I, like her mother, might be too busy to help her out. It seemed like an impossible double bind. I said to Ms. D. that I felt that whatever I said would not be what she wanted to hear: either I would remove her liberty and make her decisions for her, or I was unavailable to do so. We could both only fail.

By acknowledging this futility in the transference, Ms. D. began to experience the same sense of abandonment that she felt from her mother and began to think about this in relation to her relationship to her children. By idealising an emotionally available mother object, she had overidentified with the unconscious father object with which she had dissociated. She came to understand that she had projected her own drama onto her children, who then experienced what she regarded as loving affection as anxiety-provoking control. Remembering was not, therefore, an instant pathway to working through here: the 'ghosts in this nursery' were Ms. D.'s unheard cries and vulnerability – *the ghost/internal object had survived by its viral sense of expediency and generated relational experiences which ensured the survival of a family curse of either impingement or complete absence*. Despite Ms. D.'s own desperate need for tenderness, the curse had continued to deprive her of it by unconsciously alienating her children. Thus, the 'gap' she filled with her 'availability', ironically, would have been better left open. By making links with her ghosts, Ms. D. could now understand that there was nothing really 'wrong' with her parenting style but that there were ghosts of her own childhood which needed to be laid to rest. Through understanding her own rage at her feelings of abandonment by her mother and suffocation by her impinging father, she could then affectively experience her own care and tenderness for her children and feel compassion for them once again.

Intercultural Hauntings

As the *Ghosts in the Nursery* paper and this brief case illustration demonstrate, working through the trauma of our own childhoods and naming its affects enables us to experience feelings of care and tenderness for others. Nevertheless, due to the horrific nature of certain aspects of intergenerational trauma, this may be impossible for some. Psychotherapists have spoken about intergenerational trauma for many years, but as Lennox Thomas rightly asserts, there is a serious shortfall from an intercultural and racial perspective, and this was thrown in stark relief with the death of George Floyd and the subsequent events in 2020 (Thomas, 2019, p. 138). Enforced separation is an important aspect of the intergenerational trauma of slavery, the latter of which has come to be known as 'post-traumatic slavery syndrome' (Thomas, 2019, p. 139). This syndrome leads to a veiling of the self, resulting in what Thomas calls a 'proxy' identity which is forged to protect the subject from the projections of a racist society within which she is trying to integrate (Thomas, 2019).

Recognition Trauma

One of the foundational and most difficult aspects of working interculturally is recognition of what has taken place and one's symbolic part in it. Recognition trauma is a concept which

> identifies the process that both black and white people go through when emerging from being silenced about racism. It describes the awakening of hurtful experiences, which sometimes evokes feelings of guilt, shame, hurt and anger.
>
> (McKenzie-Mavinga, 2011)

Recognition trauma, therefore, must account for transference, countertransference, and pre-transference. The painful feelings associated with such hurtful experiences may make it difficult for client and therapist, as they may re-enact unthinking or limbic victim-oppressor dynamics associated with the paranoid-schizoid position. The persecutory guilt of the latter serves only as an obstacle which closes down therapeutic action and is therefore experienced by each member of the dyad as a *phantom* silencing. As a result of the transferences, such as those created by post-traumatic slavery syndrome, clients may find it re-traumatising to take responsibility for bringing it into the consulting room, and if the therapist does not acknowledge it either, paranoid-schizoid dynamics are likely to ensue. This is particularly the case when white therapists do not acknowledge their own awareness of what they may represent to a client of colour in the transference. This consequently may be experienced by the client as a re-enactment of intergenerational trauma – *collusion* in concealment, a turning of the blind eye, or even deceit.

If client and therapist in intercultural dyads are, however, able to begin to recognise the trauma and their personal and symbolic relations to it, there is the possibility of moving from persecution and hurt to mourning. I would argue, therefore, that as therapists, we need to pay particular attention to our affective responses to racial content in sessions and to bring these to supervision and personal therapy as they emerge. Ellis compares the process of recognition trauma to moving from the paranoid-schizoid to the depressive position (2019, p. 75).

> Once unconscious material related to race begins to surface, there is then a recognition of an awakening of the hurt related to racism as a victim or as a witness.

In order for this shift to take place, it is important that therapists facilitate a 'thinking space' where 'thoughtful objects' can be fostered to tolerate the persecutory emotions associated with discussing race (Lowe, 2014, p. 11). In order to do this – as McKenzie-Mavinga asserts – for the process of recognition trauma to take place, therapists need to be attuned to their own 'ancestral baggage' and its affects. Here, the concept of 'pre-transference' plays an important role, as both clients and therapists bring a range of conscious and unconscious preconceptions to the table. For white therapists, this means acknowledging the privileges gained from an unequal system to the detriment of people of colour. This includes understanding that

> interpersonal experiences, internalized objects, senses of self, and relational patterns that constitute transferences are culturally shaped.
>
> (Seeley, 2000, p. 210)

Ignoring these crucial cultural aspects compounds the aforementioned dissociated self-states (alien/proxy self) which contribute to an *erasure of wounded, enraged parts of the self*, which are then replaced by the phantoms of secrecy and silence.

Another important aspect of working interculturally – and particularly relevant for this book – is working with differences related to spiritual and religious subjectivity. Abernethy and Lancia, identify two forms of what they call 'religiocultural transference' (1998, p. 283):

> Interreligious transference may emerge when the patient perceives that the therapist and the patient have different religious backgrounds. Intrareligious transference may occur when the patient perceives that therapist and patient have similar religious backgrounds.

These two transferences each have their countertransference counterpart. Given the secularist materialism that pervades much of Western psychotherapy and the pejorative line that has been drawn between spiritual, magical, and religious phenomenology and omnipotent mental functioning, where there is interreligious transference, clients may avoid speaking about their beliefs altogether for fear of being perceived as a 'magical thinker'. In cases of intrareligious transference, there may be a tendency to symbiosis or the avoidance of difference. In either case, clients may be deprived of healing as a result of contemptuous rationalism or denial of individual agency and subjectivity. The dismissal of difference through symbiotic denial of its existence or 'Western' logocentric forms of rationalisation is likely to encourage situations where clients are unconsciously forced to accept an 'alien' or 'proxy' self rather than benefitting from a therapeutic relationship which helps them to discover what is hidden in the crypt of the unconscious.

Concluding Comments

This chapter has illustrated some mechanisms that contribute to the 'ancestral curse' of intergenerational trauma. We have seen the way in which defence mechanisms may also be inherited by successive generations, such as in cases of the phantom secret, the isolated affects in the nursery, the dissociative defences of disorganised attachment, identification with the aggressor, and the 'alien' self. This applies to trauma related to the Holocaust, slavery, racism, and neglect caused by socio-economic inequality. As the work of Abraham and Torok demonstrates, the phantom of intergenerational trauma consists of beta elements, which are transmitted through nonverbal suggestion or implication and become part of the unconscious phantasies of the primary curse: like dissociation, these internal objects are inimical to mentalisation. The research in this chapter importantly shows that the intergenerational curse survives with a viral expediency, thriving on the currency of paranoid-schizoid internal objects which provide families with a *jouissance* (Lacan, 1981) of masochistic gratification, all of which obstruct alpha function and are also likely to present themselves in transference enactments (Bion, 1984).

Psychotherapy, of course, may never fully reveal what the 'actual' trauma is, yet if the therapist is able to demonstrate that she is not afraid of the phantom and can instil an atmosphere of intersubjective safety within the dyad, this will then enable clients to feel that they may safely express the guilt, shame, or rage that is associated with the trauma. In order to address the limbic nature of dissociation, however, research into psychotherapy suggests that facilitating the safe expression of these somato-sensory aspects is also a core part of the treatment, and 'cognitive' or symptom-related approaches will fall short of enabling clients towards reflective functioning and an embodied recognition of what has taken place (Van der Hart and Horst, 1989). We have also seen that post-slavery syndrome has become a phantom which has left a traumatising gap. Until very recently, discussions of racial trauma have been marginalised in psychotherapeutic discourse, an indicator of an ancestral curse of prejudice.

Note

1 This appears to be based on Anna Freud's version of this defence, as the subject 'impersonates' the aggressor. See Freud (2011). Ferenczi also used this concept, though it differs from Anna Freud's formulation. This is set out in Chapter 6.

References

Abernethy, A. D. and Lancia, J. J. (1998). Religion and the psychotherapeutic relationship. transferential and countertransferential dimensions. *The Journal of Psychotherapy Practice and Research*, 7(4): 281–289.

Abraham, N., Torok, M. (1994). Rand, N. T. (Trans/ ed.) *The Shell and the Kernel: Renewals of Psychoanalysis*. Chicago: University of Chicago Press.

Bion, W. (1984). *Learning from Experience*. London: Maresfield Library.

Brothers, D. (2013). Traumatic attachments: Intergenerational trauma, dissociation, and the analytic relationship. *International Journal of Psychoanalytic Self Psychology*, 9(1): 3–15.

Ellis, E. (2019). Finding Our Voice Across the Black/white Divide: Race Issues in Therapy. In B. Ababio and R. Littlewood (eds), *Intercultural Therapy*. London and New York: Routledge.

Fairbairn, R. (1943 [1952]). The Repression and the Return of Bad Objects (with Special Reference to the 'War Neuroses'). In W. R. Fairbairn (ed), *Psychoanalytic Studies of the Personality*. London: Routledge and Kegan Paul.

Fonagy, P. (1999). The transgenerational transmission of holocaust trauma. *Attachment & Human Development*, 1(1): 92–114.

Fonagy, P., Steele, M., Moran, G., Steele, H. and Higgitt, A. (1993). Measuring the ghost in the nursery: An empirical study of the relation between parents' mental representations of childhood experiences and their infants' security of attachment. *Journal of the American Psychoanalytic Association*, 41(4): 957–989.

Fraiberg, S., Adelson, E. and Shapiro, V. (1975*)*. Ghosts in the nursery. *Journal of American Academy of Child Psychiatry*, 14(3): 387–421.

Freud, A. (2011). *The Ego and the Mechanisms of Defence*. London: Karnac Books.

Freud, S. (1919). The 'Uncanny'. In Freud, A., Strachey, A., Strachey, J, and Tyson A. (Eds.), *The Standard Edition of the Complete Psychological Works of Sigmund Freud, Volume XVII (1917–1919): An Infantile Neurosis and Other Works*. London: Hogarth Press and the Institute of Psychoanalysis, pp. 217–256.

Lacan, J. (1981). *Book XI the Four Fundamentals of Psychoanalysis*. London: W.R. Norton.

Liotti, G. (2004). Trauma, dissociation, and disorganized attachment: Three strands of a single braid. *Psychotherapy: Theory, Research, Practice*, Freud, A., Strachey, A., Strachey, J, and Tyson A. (Eds.), *Training*, 41(4): 472–486.

Lowe, F. (2014). Thinking Space: The Model. In *Thinking Space: Promoting Thinking about Race, Culture, and Diversity in Psychotherapy and beyond* (The Tavistock Clinic Series). London: Karnac, pp. 11–34.

McKenzie-Mavinga, L. (2011). The concept of recognition trauma and emerging from the hurt of racism. *Black, African and Asian Therapy Network*, September. www.baatn.org.uk/Documents/Training

Prager, J. (2016). Disrupting the Intergenerational Transmission of Trauma: Recovering Humanity, Repairing Generations. In P. Gobodo-Madikizela (ed), *Breaking Intergenerational Cycles of Repetition: A Global Dialogue on Historical Trauma and Memory* (1st edn). London: Verlag Barbara Budrich, pp. 12–26.

Schwab, G. (2010). *Haunting Legacies: Violent Histories and Transgenerational Trauma*. New York: Columbia University Press.

Seeley, K. M. (2000). *Cultural Psychotherapy: Working with Culture in the Clinical Encounter*. Northvale: Jason Aronson.

Thomas, L. (2019). Intercultural Therapy and Generationally Transmitted Trauma. In B. Ababio and R. Littlewood (eds), *Intercultural Therapy*. London and New York: Routledge.

Van der Hart, O. and Horst, R. (1989). The dissociation theory of Pierre Janet. *Journal of Traumatic Stress*, 2: 397–412.

Van der Kolk, B. A. (2015). *The Body Keeps the Score: Brain, Mind, and Body in the Healing of Trauma*. New York: Penguin Books.

Wallin David, J. (2007). *Attachment in Psychotherapy*. New York: Guildford Press.

Chapter 6

Imposters of Love

Introjection and Identification

Introduction

Building upon the origins of the curse position set out in previous chapters, I now develop this further with an important exploration of the psychic processes of introjection and identification. These meta-psychological processes offer important differing epistemological avenues into thinking about how and what is 'taken in' for the curse position to take hold and then recur. These different perspectives of 'taking in' (introjection) and 'taking on' (identification) are elaborated upon through the associated theories of Ferenczi's 'teratoma' and Klein's 'terrifying figures', which offer new perspectives on the uncanny double and – combined with the fairy lore myths of the 'changeling' and 'glamour' – shed important light on superego functioning in the curse position and its relation to *the symbolic spectacle* and imposter syndrome. These perspectives are illustrated Doris Lessing's *The Fifth Child* novella and a clinical vignette.

Introjection

In introjection, bad objects are 'taken into' the ego and become the objects of unconscious phantasies (Ferenczi, 1994a, p. 47). This describes the child's omnipotent phantasy that she can control and mediate her anxieties through primitive defences. However, such phantasies can be quickly undone through situations where 'trigger' affects – which Jung called the 'complexes' – are activated and associated with events that originally led to the introjection (Jung et al., 2014, p. 119). Ferenczi agrees that introjections, like complexes, are part of psychic life for us all, and the more aware we are of our introjections, the healthier we become.

From Introjection to Identification

For Freud, identification comes before object love; it offers the *possibility* of mutuality and 'may signify love' (1917, p. 250). Importantly, in narcissistic identification, 'object-cathexis' is renounced, yet in hysteria it persists (ibid.). These views expressed in *Mourning and Melancholia* provide an epistemological bridge from Freud to Ferenczi and the latter's concept of the 'identification with the aggressor'

DOI: 10.4324/9781003168027-7

set out in his 1933 paper *Confusion of Tongues*. Ferenczi asserts that those with relational trauma are compelled

> to subordinate themselves like automata to the will of the aggressor, to divine each one of his desires and to gratify these; completely oblivious of themselves.
>
> (Ferenczi, 1988, p. 202)

The child's defensive response to the trauma is to therefore subtract the aggressive object from the external world by introjecting it, a process which is propelled by the phantasy of the 'previous situation of tenderness' which is maintained by a 'traumatic trance' (Ferenczi, 1988, p. 202). Winnicott's work on omnipotence is germane here:

> infancy is the period in which the capacity for gathering external factors into the area of the infant's omnipotence is in process of formation. The ego support of the maternal care enables the infant to live and develop in spite of his being not yet able to control, or to feel responsible for, what is good and bad in the environment.
>
> (1960, p. 585)

The phantasy that the child can preserve the tenderness through the 'traumatic trance' at this stage of omnipotence sets the scene for subsequent phantasies of possessing 'special' powers to understand and attune to the needs and desires of the other through recurring hypnotic identifications. This is how – unbeknownst to the child – the trance has rendered her a lifeless 'automaton', as her traumatic experiences remain dissociated. However, she has introjected and therefore *identifies with* the relational grammar of aggression and/or seduction, the *imposters of love*. She has also introjected her caretakers' disowned guilt, leaving her feeling 'innocent and culpable at the same time' (Ferenczi, 1988, p. 202). The painful and maddening incompatibility of these affects cause the child to repeatedly seek out the anesthetising properties of the trance and are therefore the basis of the seductive appeal of psychopathology. The disavowed guilt of the aggressor in identification and the absence of genuinely caring and tender object relations at the stage of omnipotence all also contribute towards a persecutory superego, which will be covered in more detail later in this chapter.

As already noted above, the identification with the aggressor drives all identifications and phantasies hereafter, which 'can become habitual and can lead to masochism, chronic hypervigilance, and other personality distortions' (Frankel, 2002, p. 101). This masochistic hypervigilance is a key aspect of the curse position where the individual scans objects for omens of misfortune which are then introjected, driven by the phantasy in the primary curse that they can be managed or controlled, yet are instead just more grist to the mill of self-persecution.

The 'Teratoma'

As we have seen from Chapter 2, Ferenczi shared Freud's interest in the occult and in the *doppelgänger* through which he developed his concept of the 'teratoma'. For Freud, the uncanny double presents developmental confusions and distortions of identity, but Ferenczi's 'teratoma' double is parasitic, and

> harbours in a hidden part of its body fragments of a twin-being which has never developed. No reasonable person would refuse to surrender such a teratoma to the surgeon's knife, if the existence of the whole individual were threatened.
>
> (Ferenczi, 1994b, p. 123)

The ontological evolution of the double from a Freudian to a Ferenczian mutation serves to illustrate the qualitative difference between neurotic and traumatic reality: where Freud's double represents the denial of death, Ferenczi's 'teratoma' is a psychic parasite which, although arrested in development, dominates object relations thereafter. Ferenczi's analogy of the surgeon's knife illustrates the way in which the attempted 'extraction' of hurt aspects of the self by therapists may threaten the very existence of the client and thus remain effectively inaccessible to treatment.

Klein

Notwithstanding the radical difference in Klein's approach from her former analyst's, Ferenczi's influence on her theories is evident – particularly regarding introjection, splitting, identification, and projection – despite scant references to his work by Klein and her followers.[1] For Klein, like Ferenczi, projection and introjection are ongoing processes: In *Our Adult World and Its Roots in Infancy*, she writes,

> I have spoken of introjection and the external world and have hinted that this process continues throughout life. Whenever we admire and love somebody – we also *take something of them into ourselves* and our deepest attitudes are shaped by such experiences. In the one case it enriches us and becomes a foundation for precious memories; in the other case we sometimes feel that the outer world is spoilt for us and the inner world is therefore impoverished.
>
> (Klein, 1997b, p. 256; italics my own)

The feeling that the outer world has been spoilt is pertinent to the next quotation in the same paper, where Klein continues in a more radical vein, her own metapsychology now distinct with its depressive/persecutory dialectical focus:

> However, much depends, even in the infant, on the ways in which external influences are interpreted and assimilated by the child, and this in turn largely

depends on how strongly destructive impulses and persecutory and depressive anxieties are operative.

(ibid.)

Here, the emphasis is on the endogenous position of the child and whether she operates from a persecutory 'paranoid-schizoid'[2] or 'depressive' anxiety. In the former, love and hate are split, and destructive impulses reign; in the latter, she is able to seek reparation through anxieties associated with guilt (Klein, 1997a, pp. 253–255). Despite Klein's frequent use of the epistemology of introjection and projection, in terms of identification, it is the latter which, of course, she is most associated with:

It seems that the processes underlying projective identification operate already in the earliest relation to the breast. The 'vampire-like' sucking, the scooping out of the breast, develop in the infant's phantasy into making his way into the breast and further into the mother's body.

(Klein, 1997d, p. 69)

Here, the child expels the aggressive 'badness' which she is unable to tolerate into a phantasised part object which she then re-introjects as persecutory anxiety in the paranoid-schizoid position. Interestingly, Klein uses the vampire as a metaphor to describe a *parasitic* 'scooping out', though milk rather than blood is the target. This greedy kind of introjection evokes Gambian *buwaa* and *ukuñaabe* witches who are believed capable of '"sucking out" their life force until the victims get very sick and die' (O'Neill et al., 2015, p. 5).

A Wolof marabout[3] explains,

You know if you put the insect in a small container with a groundnut, it will suck away all the liquid contained in the seed. That is the same way that the witches operate.

(ibid.)

This 'scooping out' also calls to mind a relational dynamic between the witch and his/her demon 'familiar' in European folklore. Emma Wilby defines the demon familiar as 'any spirit which enters into a relationship with a witch and gives her magical assistance' and therefore is reminiscent of the *daimon* introduced in earlier chapters (2005, p. 58). Importantly, Wilby points out that during the witch trials of the 16th and 17th centuries in the UK, the church and the state made no distinction between maleficent and benign magic, and this also applied to helpful or harmful familiars: all were essentially deemed to be evil[4] (2005, p. 55). In a confession taken from one witchcraft trial in 1582, Margery Sammon claimed that she had been instructed by her mother how to tend to her toad familiars – called Tom and Robin – with the chilling injunction: *If thou dost not give them milk, they will suck of thy blood*, which perhaps may serve as a metaphor for the pressures on the mother – and indeed the psychotherapist – to gratify (Wilby, 2005, p. 109).

The Fifth Child

Where for Ferenczi the parasite becomes a split-off part of the psyche, for Klein the child itself is parasitic, relentlessly demanding the breast. In her novel *The Fifth Child*, Doris Lessing brilliantly illustrates the dreadful consequences for a mother of being the recipient of an infant's aggression. Harriet and David Lovatt meet in the swinging 60s in London, a time of burgeoning liberalism, as the staid conservatism of the previous decade fades. Yet the newlyweds identify much more with the humdrum idealism of yore and move to a large house in a commuter town to start a family. Despite the largely cloying and symbiotic idealism on display in the preliminary stages of the couple's relationship, a tenebrous undertow is hinted at early on. There is a menacing, and demonic aspect which Harriet sees in David, indicating an omen of things to come.

There is a clear avoidance of the 'bad' in the couple – an implicit terror of things getting *spoiled*: they seek to avoid listening to the news broadcasts on the radio, as if they wish to be insulated from a threatening real. There is also a shared omnipotence as they gratuitously phantasise about their miraculous capacity to succeed in getting other people together that are close to them and making them happy. Nevertheless, paradise is soon lost as the couple's use of idealism as a means of shoring up persecutory anxieties begins to crack. Harriet attributes the birth of her sister and brother-in-law's baby daughter with Down syndrome to the result of their arguments, as if it were a divine punishment. Harriet then begins to display a superstitious tendency which irks her husband. This persecutory anxiety in Harriet points to a dreaded object in the couple which they both fear they will give birth to and is defended against by displacement in her and denial in him. David shows a rationalist hypocrisy towards what he believes are Harriet's hysterical tendencies yet displays his own superstitious leanings, where – couched in macho jocularity – he makes reference more than once to the fertile properties of the bedroom.

Despite some difficult pregnancies for Harriet, the births of four children go otherwise smoothly. This is, of course, until Ben arrives – child number five. Ben appears to be a humanoid, possessed by a demonic spirit, and from the uterine stage is already kicking violently inside Harriet's womb. Harriet now experiences the horror of a concrete confirmation of the previously dreaded object. She is now in excruciating pain and begins to have dark fantasies about a satanic creature in her womb. When Ben is finally born following an agonising struggle, the reality confirms her worst suspicions, as he looks more like a troll or goblin than a baby. Ben is at one point referred to as a changeling, which also refers to the idea in fairy lore that a child has been replaced by one from fairyland, which is discussed in detail in the subsequent section.

When Ben begins breastfeeding, the reader is confronted by horrifying imagery, highly evocative of a Kleinian baby, as he violently sucks and bites on his mother's breasts and nipples. It is not long before David and other members of the family convince Harriet to send Ben away as his aggressive behaviour becomes overwhelming and his siblings are now terrified of him. David then threatens Harriet with an ultimatum: she must either choose Ben or the rest of the family.

Harriet agrees to send Ben away to a care home for delinquent children but is then unable to live with her conscience and decides to visit him. She is horrified to discover he has been cruelly neglected, which leaves Ben severely traumatised. Harriet is overcome with horror at Ben's treatment and takes him back to the family home. Ben then continues to live with the family for the rest of the novella, but the consequences of his continued anti-social behaviour are devastating. His siblings gradually relocate to boarding schools or to live with relatives, and the Lovatts grow increasingly distant from one another. Harriet believes that the breakdown of the family serves as a punishment for their desire for happiness. Despite David's attempts to show Harriet that her thought processes are more at home in the 16th century witch trials than in 20th century suburbia, she is now at the mercy of the secondary curse, where the superego comprises entirely the persecutory phantasies of the primary curse. David notices that Harriet's masochistic imagination is also redolent of the malevolent gods of the archaic unconscious, yet as he becomes increasingly desperate, he also begins to waiver and have similar persecutory thoughts that someone or something *has it in for them.*

The couple fail to see that these same arcane and cruel gods are those trolls and goblins of deep time that they have located in Ben. Their continuing disowned aggression and inability to mourn their ideal child leads to a persecutory guilt from which they cannot recover. Ben, as the 'weird child' par excellence, is *fated* to never belong, and he is even denied subjectivity altogether. If we were to treat this as a piece of meta-fiction, this in itself would be Ben's deepest trauma. There is no insight into Ben's mind available to the reader – implicitly, it is as if, as the goblin child, he does not deserve one – aside from glimpses into a vulnerability that has been overlooked, even debased by 'normal' people. The Lovatts themselves and their children – including Ben – are victims not of ancient and merciless gods but the collapse of the defences of an idealized object that is flooded by persecutory tides as the curse position takes hold:

> A very deep split between the two aspects of the object indicates that it is not the good and bad object that are being kept apart but an idealized and an extremely bad one. So deep and sharp a division reveals that destructive impulses, envy, and persecutory anxiety are very strong and that idealization serves mainly as a defence against these emotions.
>
> (Klein, 1997a, p. 191)

When one is flooded by the persecutory imagination of the primary curse, recourse to the paranoid-schizoid position is the only option: Harriet at one stage appears psychotically overwhelmed by phantasies from the archaic unconscious as she states her belief that Ben is not human and that his diminutive relatives hail from subterranean places. This terror of an arcane, underground civilisation of 'little people' recalls Arthur Machen's description in *The Novel of the Black Seal*:

> Nothing they have in common with me save the face, and the customs of humanity are wholly strange to them and they hate the sun. They hiss rather than speak; their voices are harsh, and not to be heard without fear.
>
> (Machen, 2011, p. 42)

Klein's 'Terrifying Figures' and the Curse Position

These 'little people' may be the returning of the repressed spirits of the archaic unconscious or wounded elements of a pre-symbolic self, deprived of language: the remnants of the primary curse. These split-off proto representations of a traumatised infancy now roam the deepest unconscious like the damned of Dante's *Inferno*. Given the highly persecutory nature of the Lovatts' experience in *The Fifth Child*, it is these 'terrifying figures'[5] which transcend the usual Kleinian dialectic of good and bad objects which, at the most extreme levels of anxiety and trauma, overwhelm the ego.

> Terrifying figures make themselves felt when internal or external pressure is extreme. People who are on the whole stable – and that means that they have firmly established their good object and therefore are closely identified with it – can overcome this intrusion of the *deeper unconscious* into their ego and regain their stability. In neurotic, and still more in psychotic individuals, the struggle against such dangers threatening from the deep layers of the unconscious is to some extent constant and part of their instability or their illness.
>
> (Klein, 1997c, p. 243; italics my own)

Kleinian analyst Ronald Britton postulates that the objects which reside in this deeper unconscious are 'supernatural' and

> form the basis for beliefs about heaven and hell not normally experienced but hypothesised in religions and art, except by some individuals as visions such as Joan of Arc or William Blake.
>
> (Britton, 2015, p. 18)

Britton therefore makes an intriguing connection between Klein's 'deeper unconscious' and mythopoetic consciousness. From this perspective, the 'terrifying figures' evoke Spare's notion of 'intrusive familiars' – agents of magical consciousness – described in Chapter 4 (Staley, 2011).

According to Klein – based on her observation of infants – the objects of the deeper unconscious are the result of introjection – they are pushed into these deeper strata and cannot therefore be integrated into the ego in the same way as the superego. What Klein does not really explain, however, is what determines the particularly punitive nature of these introjected 'terrifying objects'. Ferenczi here provides a useful additional perspective, emphasising developmental trauma as a causative factor:

> if the shocks increase in number during the development of the child, the number and the various kinds of splits in the personality increase too, and soon it becomes extremely difficult to maintain contact without confusion with all the fragments, each of which behaves as a separate personality yet does not know of even the existence of the others. Eventually it may arrive at a state which – continuing the picture of fragmentation – one would be justified in calling *atomization*.
>
> (1988, p. 205)

For Ferenczi, *atomization* is the result of traumatic 'shocks'. This atomization is what gives the 'little people' of the deepest layers of the unconscious their independence and dissociative unawareness of one another. Each is an independent but destructive entity emerging from the psychic magma: warring goblins, fairies, and imps of the mind. These entities manifest as an 'imaginary real': they present as images yet are agonisingly non-symbolic (Žižek, 2001). It is these elements under times of inner or outer stress which arrive from the unconscious and wreak havoc on object relations. Whether these entities are part of the superego or operate independently of it is, however, debatable. For Klein, those with sufficiently robust ego strength will withstand such attacks from the 'terrifying figures', but this becomes an increasingly vulnerable continuum between neurosis and schizophrenia, where, in the latter state of mind, they are indistinguishable from the superego. For fear of making generalisations about psychopathology in relation to the 'terrifying figures', I will restrict my view to the curse position. Briefly then, states of psychic pressure or duress – caused by internal or external activations of anxiety – trigger the primary curse, which the ego experiences as a highly persecutory conscience. Due to the flooding of the non-symbolising imaginary real into the ego, the prohibitive part of the superego is perceived by the ego as inimical and persecutory, rather than as protecting its good objects – as in symbolic function – and is therefore a key element of the secondary curse. This interaction between the 'terrifying figures' and the superego in the curse position is now explored further in relation to the folklore of the 'changeling'.

The Changeling

In fairy lore, changelings are children who have been substituted by fairies for a human child who has been kidnapped to live in fairyland. Reasons for the kidnap are various and beyond the scope of this paper, though folklorist Katharine Briggs provides a succinct summary:

> The children seem to have been changed for a double reason, both to recruit the fairy stock with a human admixture and to give the substituted changeling a chance of human nurture.
>
> (Briggs, 1957, p. 274)

It has been argued that changeling myths arose as a socio-cultural response to children who were considered 'abnormal' and had physical or intellectual disabilities (Lyle, 1970; Schoon Eberly, 1988). The myth connects with Christian beliefs in the 16th and 17th centuries in the British Isles which regarded disabled children as a result of 'divine chastisement' for a mother's sin (Schoon Eberly, 1988, p. 60). As a result of such beliefs, children – and in some cases adults – were abused and even killed (ibid.). These responses to the 'abnormal' raise important questions of how we, as therapists, respond to the abnormal or deformed: the 'teratoma'. The prefix *tera-* also derives from the Greek *teras*, meaning monster:

> The ancient history of teratology does not teach us much about the origin, prevention, or treatment of congenital malformation; but it tells us a great deal about the human mind and its reactions to unexplained phenomena. If an abnormal child is born to a family or a tribe, [a person] insists upon an explanation.
>
> (Warkany, quoted in Schoon Eberly, 1988, p. 59)

As we have seen in earlier chapters, the incapacity of humans to accept random chance as an acceptable explanation for uncanny misfortune and where the monstrous 'tera' appears in place of the idealised can result in devastating consequences of neglect and abuse. The pain that is caused by the removal of the 'teratoma' and the changeling may serve as metaphors for the tragic sacrifices that are made by the vulnerable in the service of alleviating the terrors of deformity in those who are supposed to take care of them. This also, of course, applies to working with difference in the transference. I now focus on another example from *The Fifth Child* to illustrate this point.

Although *The Fifth Child* is not a strictly faithful allegory of the changeling myth, it contains important aspects of it. Firstly, there is Harriet's interpretation of the birth of her sister's child with Down syndrome, Amy, as a 'divine' punishment. Although there is no mention of a religious affiliation in Harriet, this is an early indicator of her implicit identification with the aggressor (evoking changeling lore and church doctrine), as Harriet cannot envisage that Amy's arrival can be received with tenderness, *only horror*. It is no surprise, then, that when Ben is born, he is perceived as if he were an evil changeling who has cruelly taken the place of a wished-for baby and is consequently sent away to a care facility where he is, at best, cruelly neglected and, at worst, traumatically abused.

Symbolic Folly

The metaphor of the changeling also illustrates an important relationship between the births of Amy and, subsequently, Ben in terms of their impact on Harriet's unconscious processes and illustrates an important aspect of the curse position. Through introjective identification, Amy's birth activates the primary curse in Harriet as she perceives the child with Down syndrome as a portent of her own future punishment. As part of Harriet's introjected phantasy, Amy becomes a bad omen, as the primary element of the curse position imbues present symbols with significance and power *as if they contain the 'actual' symbolic portent of the curse: they become living things in one's mind*. Yet crucially, such omens are part of an imaginary 'lure' (Lacan, 1981, p. 100). The subject – fuelled by the terror of the deeper unconscious – is therefore bewitched into perceiving the object as the symbol of a curse, creating a *symbolic folly* – what Zizek calls a 'spectral supplement' (2001, p. 93) – Fisher's 'something where there should be nothing' (2016, p. 67). Crucially though, in the symbolic folly of the curse position, the unconscious uses the symbolising capacity of the ego against itself by *pretending* to represent something it is not. It is this pretence which stems from the trauma of the introjection and identification with the aggressor that is the kernel of the symbolic folly, and this is what leads the subject to feel that she is herself an imposter, a clown, and a fool.

The Glamour

We can also think about this alluring compulsion in folkloric terms. The 'glamour' of fairly lore further illustrates the temporal distortion of the curse position. This 'glamour' is a bewitching spell that fairies place humans under, and importantly, it also alters perception of temporal reality: the timelessness of the unconscious is then also experienced as if it were part of secondary process. Harriet appears to be under the 'glamour' of a fairy time slip when pregnant with Ben as the presence of 'intrusive familiars' distort temporal reality.

Here, Harriet is fully under the 'glamour' of the primary curse; her 'terrifying figures' have fully colonised her superego, and the resulting persecutory phantasies create a weird, alienating dissonance from those around her. When Ben is born, he becomes one of these frightening chimeras incarnate, a living embodiment of the 'teratoma'.

This example from Harriet elucidates the way in which the 'terrifying figures' of the curse position function as changeling doubles which emerge from the deep unconscious and hijack the superego. The overwhelming terror that the ego experiences means that the superego's function of benign prohibition becomes self-attacking. Under the 'glamour' of the primary curse, the subject has unknowingly exchanged her benign conscience for a changeling aggressor who implicitly 'knows best': the changeling superego is given credit where it is not due – for being nasty. This is a significant contributor to a pull towards sado-masochistic relationships.

In fairy lore, the changelings which replace the infants are sometimes said to have 'wizened' faces, as they are elderly in fairy time. Human parents, though, are duped by the 'glamour' into thinking they are their own children. This aspect of lore evokes Ferenczi's concept of the 'wise child':

> The fear of the uninhibited, almost mad adult changes the child, so to speak, into a psychiatrist and, in order to become one and to defend himself against dangers coming from people without self-control, he must know how to identify himself completely with them. Indeed, it is unbelievable how much we can still learn from our wise children, the neurotics.
>
> (Ferenczi, 1994b], p. 165)

The 'wise child', then, is born of the madness of adults which he has been forced to introject and identify with: his 'wizened' face is testament to the toll of life lived with trauma.

Clinical Vignette

Ms. S., a woman in her 20s, had been in therapy for several months. Her mother suffered from bi-polar disorder and had been verbally and sometimes physically abusive since she was a child. Although her mother would apologise for her behaviour the next day – as it was always framed in terms of her mother's persecutory guilt rather than genuine remorse – Ms. S. always felt that it was 'all about her' and left her feeling guilty. Although Ms. S. had fond memories of playing football in the park with her father as a child, he was a heavy drinker and would often argue with her mother in front of Ms. S. and her younger sister, which would become more severe when he was drunk. He was also away often with work, which Ms. S.'s mother resented, and she suspected him of infidelity. Ms. S.'s father would also treat her more as a friend than a daughter and, when drunk, would speak about his desire to leave her mother and tell her that he had lied to her mother about his whereabouts. Although Ms. S. hated to think about these conversations, she said that they made her feel important at the time, as if only she could make her father feel better.

Ms. S. dreaded her father being away, as this always meant her mother's abusive behaviour towards her and her sister would worsen. She had done well academically at primary school, where her teachers really encouraged her obvious imaginative capacity, and she felt she had talent for art. When Ms. S.'s parents' marriage began to break down in her teens, the quality of her academic work declined considerably, and this is when her bulimia began.

Although Ms. S. had always enjoyed art at school and wanted to pursue this as a potential career, in the end, she chose to study accountancy at university, as she knew that was her mother's preference. Ms. S. now worked as a bookkeeper for a blue-chip firm and felt that it was 'soulless'; she was now in crisis and had recently started bingeing and purging food daily. She said that she felt like an imposter at work, as she had never genuinely been interested in finance as a career, and although she would have liked a job which she considered more creative and meaningful, she said that she was too old to change now. When Ms. S. perceived her friends to be flourishing in their careers and relationships, this became a confirmation of her inherent misfortune. Ms. S. said that she felt controlled by a mean inner critical voice which repeatedly told her that she wasn't a 'normal human being' and was useless or stupid.

Ms. S. usually arrived punctually for her sessions, but one evening she had been held up by public transport and arrived around 10 minutes late. She had texted me to let me know, but when she arrived, was obviously anxious and apologised to me profusely. When I replied that I understood that this was a situation beyond her control, Ms. S. then smiled as if she wanted to portray a feeling of relief, but she remained sitting on the edge of the chair with her coat on and

appeared quite anxious. Ms. S. then quickly asked me how I was and if I had
had a good weekend. I was aware of the way Ms. S.'s trauma history impacted
on her unconscious phantasies and object relations, and I therefore did not wish
to respond in a way which she would experience as punitive. However, I did not
want to make a concrete disclosure because a) this would have closed things
down and b) I felt some anxiety about the question, as if there were something
quite intrusive yet insincere about it. I therefore decided instead to say that I appreciated that she wished to know but thought it would be most helpful to think
together about what this meant to her. Initially, Ms. S. seemed irritated by this
and said that it was 'normal' for people to ask one another how they are and told
me that she felt it was 'weird' that she only ever spoke about herself in therapy
and that I didn't disclose anything. I agreed that it was indeed 'weird', but this
was a therapy session where we might explore 'weird' things, and, as she didn't
usually ask me how my weekend was, I wondered if she had been worried that I
was angry with her for not being on time and that this had been a way of finding
out. Ms. S. initially said that she didn't see what I was getting at, but after taking
a moment to think about it, said that she felt like she was 'always people pleasing'
and at that point burst into tears. She then reached for a tissue to blow her nose
and let out a despondent but angry sigh which appeared to bring her some relief.
Intuitively, I suspected that Ms. S. might now be more receptive to explore what
had taken place, and after a few moments I said,

> 'I was wondering whether what you are saying about "people pleasing" con-
> nects in some way to asking me about the weekend?'
> 'How do you mean?', she asked, with a quizzical but searching expression.
> 'Well, I was wondering how you think it would make you feel if I did tell you
> about my weekend, or if I didn't'.
> She smiled and raised her eyebrows again into a quizzical expression as if
> enjoying the prospect of thinking about this. She then quickly replied,
> 'Well, I guess if you didn't tell me about your weekend, I'd understand that
> as I know that you have your boundaries you need to keep, but when I
> came late and saw your face I felt guilty so I wanted to ask you about your
> weekend to be nice I guess'. She cast her eyes downwards, as if to protect
> herself.
> After a couple more moments I asked, 'Ahh, I see. I was wondering what it
> was you saw in my face?' Aware of how vulnerable Ms. S. must have felt at
> this moment, I wanted to convey my compassion for that vulnerability by
> emphasising a gentle curiosity in my voice.
> 'Well, you looked annoyed. And so when you said that you understood the
> reason why I was late, I thought you didn't really believe me'.
> 'So being nice was a way to placate me in some way?'
> 'Yes', she answered immediately. 'It reminds me of being at home – with
> Mum, however "nice" she might have appeared, I was always on alert that
> she might turn on me – she was so mean sometimes. So the only thing I felt
> I could do was to "be nice" so that she didn't lose her rag'.

'OK. So how would you have felt if I *had* told you about my weekend?'

'Probably an over-share. [She smiled and looked a little embarrassed.] I don't really want to know. My dad always used to over-share'.

'So it seems you wanted on the one hand to "people please" by asking about my weekend in order to protect yourself from my angry feelings, but also to check out whether the boundaries were safe?'

She thought for a few moments before saying, 'I guess so, yeah. It's like I either had a dad who behaved like a mate, or a mum who was bloody scary and might switch at any moment. It felt unbearable'. She looked saddened by her summary.

'You feel now that your feelings were unbearable?'

'Yeah, and that's why I throw them up every single day'.

Discussion

It is clear Ms. S. has had to identify with hostile and narcissistic objects in lieu of care, empathy, and tenderness. As with many who have suffered relational trauma, introjecting and identifying with objects in this way is a matter of survival. Ms. S.'s self-denigration was driven by the hostile objects she has introjected that are bound up with her mother's abuse and, through the symbolic spectacle, are subsequently identified with by looking for 'signs' that she can introject, which is driven by clairvoyant hypervigilance. This introjective identification took place in the transference, driven by Ms. S.'s unconscious phantasy that there was a hostile object – a symbolic folly – which she has located in me. By re-introjecting it, the hostile folly could be placated, and she could safely return to the Ferenczian 'previous situation of tenderness' represented by the idealised football game with her father. Here, we can see the ways in which Ms. S. was unconsciously compelled to identify with the aggressor. Firstly, in the transference, by wanting to find out about my weekend, she could meet her father's narcissistic and greedy need to disregard the boundaries of care for the purposes of self-gratification. This warded off her aggressive and suspicious mother – my 'anger' at her lateness in the transference – again through the phantasised and projected return to tenderness. This transference was also driven by the part of her which identified with her father by attempting to blur the boundaries of the therapeutic relationship by asking me to tell her about my weekend. This identification was driven by Ms. S.'s omnipotent and compliant self – the 'wise child' – that *had to know what she didn't want or need to know* as a child by having to lie or hold on to information about her father. This was part of an ongoing 'bi-polar' repetition compulsion of asking about what she did not want to know, paralleling the Ferenczian innocence/culpability bind. The original association with the aggressor was – like the guilt – disowned, and the compulsion to know what one doesn't want to know therefore felt simultaneously alien yet entirely part of the self: a changeling. This compulsive bind and desire to rid herself of the changeling self was so maddening that Ms. S. could only resort to bulimia, yet the bingeing and purging were conducted under a glamour – the traumatic trance. This resulted in harm to her body which paralleled the aforementioned harm caused to the 'changeling' children by adults who could not bear their own charac-terological deformities. Another driver of the bulimia was that, under the glamour of the identification, Ms. S. unconsciously idealised the omnipotent 'wise child' but hated the split-off changeling with its old, wizened features – a terrifying and loathed object which had taken over her superego and which Ms. S. compulsively therefore attempted to spit out. All these traumatic identifications had also pro-pelled Ms. S. into a 'soulless' imposter career which she felt she could not escape and into identifying with the wizened changeling self who was 'too old' to change, despite only being in her 20s. It was also the idealisation of the wise child which created the bulimic compulsion, as there was always a pull to return to it.

The last interaction of this vignette demonstrates my aim to contain and nur-ture the good objects that Ms. S. was slowly internalising through the therapeutic relationship by ensuring that her phantasies were explored with curiosity and not sabotaged by self-disclosure. It was therefore important to be a benign superego in the transference by taking her reasons for her lateness at her word and facilitat-ing her own interpretations rather than intrusively doing that for her. Through this exchange, Ms. S. came to understand that being nice to her mother had become a means of self-sacrifice despite the symbolic folly of self-preservation: instead of warding off the demon, she had invited it. In holding the boundary, I modelled a way in which she could deal with her father's narcissistic intrusion and mother's aggression. By making the link between her parental double-bind and her bulimia, she was now beginning a process towards grieving her childhood trauma and find-ing her own language for it.

Concluding Comments

As this vignette shows, working with these kinds of identifications places a great deal of pressure on the therapist, and it is therefore quite easy to collude with the 'imposters of love' by gratifying clients too easily or responding with hostility to avoid working through important material in the transference. Through the meta-phors of the teratoma and the changeling, this chapter has shown how painful it can be to be awoken from the 'glamour' of the primary curse and to relinquish the identifications which are often omnipotent and idealised. As therapists, we there-fore need to be patient, though we are sometimes in conflict with the part of the client that wishes to stay under a glamour or induce the same in us. We also need to grapple with the terrifying figures of the changeling superego in the trans-ference which will seek to destroy interventions which lead towards working through and mourning, both of which are unconsciously perceived to be threats to the self and other. Working through and mourning are therefore achieved by standing up to the changeling superego which will incrementally re-introduce benign superego function to help clients find their own symbols of relational trauma and its effects, rather than spectacles of them. By helping clients discover their own language of trauma, psychotherapy becomes an important means of fostering liberating experiences of agency, as well as tender and loving relation-ships of mutual care.

Acknowledgement

Thank you to the *Weird Studies* podcast for their inspirational podcast on *The Fifth Child*, which was instructive for this chapter.

Notes

1 This is concordant with psychoanalytic trends of the time and Ferenczi's general ostracisation until the end of the 20th century (Soreanu, 2018, p. 3).
2 Although Klein states that the paranoid-schizoid position is dominant in the first six months of life, it is not temporally dependent, as it is a 'position' – like the curse position – which is returned to.
3 Marabouts are well-respected religious figures across West Africa who specialise in Islamic and non-Islamic spiritual matters such as prayers, healing, clairvoyance, and other rituals around life and death (O'Neill et al., 2015, p. 5).
4 Aside from the paranoid splitting of the church at this time, Wilby goes on to draw intriguing parallels between the familiars or 'helping spirits' in witchcraft and ancient cross-cultural shamanic practices.
5 I have found Raluca Soreanu's 2018 paper *The Psychic Life of Fragments: Splitting From Ferenczi to Klein* instructive in exploring with regard to Klein's 'terrifying figures'.

References

Briggs, K. M. (1957). The English fairies. *Folklore*, 68(1).
Britton, R. (2015). *Between Mind and Brain: Models of the Mind and Models in the Mind* (1st edn). London: Karnac.
Ferenczi, S. (1988). Confusion of tongues between adults and the child – The language of tenderness and of passion. *Contemporary Psychoanalysis*, 24: 196–206.
Ferenczi, S. (1994a). *First Contributions to Psychoanalysis*. London: Karnac Books.
Ferenczi, S. (1994b). *Psycho-Analysis and Education Final Contributions to Psychoanalysis*. London: Karnac Books.
Fisher, M. (2016). *The Weird and the Eerie*. London: Repeater Books.
Frankel, J. (2002). Exploring Ferenczi's concept of identification with the aggressor. *Psychoanalytic Dialogues*, 12: 101–139.
Freud, S. (1917). Mourning and Melancholia. In Freud, A., Strachey, A., Strachey, J, and Tyson A. (Eds.), *The Standard Edition of the Complete Psychological Works of Sigmund Freud* (Vol. XIV). London: The Hogarth Press and the Institute of Psychoanalysis.
Jung, C. G., Adler, G. and Hull, R. F. C. (2014). *Collected Works of C.G. Jung, Volume 16*. Princeton: Princeton University Press.
Klein, M. (1997a). Envy and Gratitude. In *Envy and Gratitude and Other Works 1946–1963* (3rd edn). London: Vintage.
Klein, M. (1997b). Our Adult World and Its Roots in Infancy. In *Envy and Gratitude and Other Works 1946–1963* (3rd edn). London: Vintage.
Klein, M. (1997c). On the Development of Mental Functioning. In *Envy and Gratitude and Other Works 1946–1963* (3rd edn). London: Vintage.
Klein, M. (1997d). Some Theoretical Conclusions Regarding the Emotional Life of the Infant. In *Envy and Gratitude and Other Works 1946–1963* (3rd edn). London: Vintage.

Lacan, J. (1981). *Book XI The Four Fundamentals of Psychoanalysis*. London: W.R. Norton.

Lyle, E. B. (1970). The Teind to Hell in TamLin, *Folklore*, 81(3): 177–181.

Machen, A. (2011). The Novel of the Black Seal. In *The White People and Other Weird Stories*. London: Penguin Books.

O'Neill, S., Gryseels, C., Dierickx, S., Mwesigwa, J., Okebe, J., d'Alessandro, U. and Peeters Grietens, K. (2015). Foul wind, spirits and witchcraft: Illness conceptions and health-seeking behaviour for Malaria in the Gambia. *Malaria Journal*, 14(167).

Schoon Eberly, S. (1988). Fairies and the folklore of disability: Changelings, hybrids and the solitary fairy. *Folklore*, 99(1): 58–77.

Shengold, L. L. (1979). Child abuse and deprivation: Soul murder. *Journal of the American Psychoanalytic Association*, 27(3): 533–59.

Soreanu, R. (2018). The psychic life of fragments: Splitting from Ferenczi to Klein. *Journal of the American Psychoanalytic*, 78: 421–444.

Staley, M. (2011). The Resurgence of Cosmic Identity. In A. O. Spare, *The Book of Pleasure (Self Love): The Psychology of Ecstasy*. London: Jerusalem Press.

Wilby, E. (2005). *Cunning Folk and Familiar Spirits: Shamanistic Visionary Tradition in Early Modern British Witchcraft and Magic*. Brighton: Sussex Academic Press.

Winnicott, D. W. (1960). The theory of the parent-infant relationship. *International Journal of Psycho-Analysis*, 41: 585–595.

Žižek, S. (2001). *On Belief*. London and New York: Routledge.

Chapter 7

Redemption & Conditionality
Fairbairn and Relational Trauma

Introduction

Building on the previous chapter's clinical themes on relational trauma, I now consider the work of the psychoanalyst Ronald Fairbairn. I demonstrate the way in which Fairbairn's theories of the 'moral defence' (1943) and 'endopsychic structures' (1944) provide us with a structural object relations theory that helps us to gain a deeper insight into the foundational elements which lead to the intractability of the repetition compulsions that stem from relational trauma. In Fairbairn's paradigm, 'bad objects' from traumatic attachments in infancy foster a 'closed system' of internal objects in which the individual becomes one's own prisoner (1994).

Fairbairn's theories have become an important influence on my clinical thinking and, moreover, in terms of the development of the curse position theory. This particularly applies to the topographic levels of relational functioning between the level of the 'primary curse' and its defensive secondary counterpart. This model draws upon Fairbairn's developmental models of primary 'libidinal attachment' and secondary defensive superego (1943). Importantly, Fairbairn shows that there is a distinctly moral form of masochism evident in developmental trauma, where parts of the self are 'renounced' in order to be 'saved' or 'redeemed', which Fairbairn calls the 'moral defence' (ibid.). The conditionality of the 'moral defence' is illustrated in 'the case of Christoph Haitzmann' – a masochistic pact between the Devil and an impoverished painter. Fairbairn's work remains highly pertinent to contemporary 'mental health' concerns today, and I therefore apply his thinking to the modern archetypes of the saviour, people pleaser, empath, and narcissist. I finally present a case illustration to demonstrate Fairbairn's theories in clinical practice and how I apply his recommendations for treatment.

Ronald Fairbairn

Ronald Fairbairn was considered an outlier in the British psychoanalytic community, partly due to his geographical remoteness from the psychoanalytical society in London but also because he was a practising Christian who attended mass throughout his life and was therefore at odds with the society's atheistic orthodoxy

DOI: 10.4324/9781003168027-8

(Hoffman and Hoffman, 2014). As a child he had attended mass at the Evangelical Free Church in Scotland with his parents, and then in middle age, due to the orthodox and puritanical nature of the free church, had joined the Anglican church (ibid.). Fairbairn's faith is pivotal to his clinical epistemology and its core departure from classical drive theory towards an 'object relations theory of the personality' (Fairbairn et al., 1994, p. 312). Judaeo-Christian currents run throughout Fairbairn's work, presenting a 'pristine' innocent child who is emotionally fractured by experience and can only be unified again through 'redemptive' love, which is a recurring theme in this chapter (Hoffman and Hoffman, 2014). Fairbairn's paradigm benefits from his direct experience of working at the Clinic for Children and Juveniles, which led him to believe that it was not the drives that were the overarching causes of psychopathology but the children's bonding to 'bad objects' resulting from dependency on abusive or neglectful caregivers (Sinason, 2014, p. 197). Importantly, in Fairbairn's structural model, it is not objects themselves which are internalised *but the ego's relationship to them as dynamic structures* (Ogden, 1983). Hence, the main epistemological emphasis is on the belief that libidinal cathexis is object based and rejects Freud's primacy of the pleasure principle.

> My point of view may, however, be stated in a word. In my opinion it is high time that psychopathological inquiry, which in the past has been successively focused, first upon impulse, and later upon the ego, should now be focused upon the object towards which impulse is directed.
>
> (Fairbairn, 1943, p. 59)

Fairbairn then goes further:

> It is difficult to see how the experience of being assaulted could afford any great measure of gratification except to the more masochistic of individuals. To the average individual such an experience is not so much guilty as simply 'bad'. It is intolerable in the main, not because it gratifies repressed impulses, but for the same reason that a child often flies panic-stricken from a stranger who enters the house. It is intolerable because a bad object is always intolerable, and a relationship with a bad object can never be contemplated with equanimity.
>
> (Fairbairn, 1943, p. 62)

This is a stirring and powerful paragraph in its repudiation of Freud's perspectives on guilt and impulse: Fairbairn's work emphasises that the trauma of developmental neglect cannot be conflated with the Oedipal guilt of prohibited drives, which is a distinctly different experience with a distinct outcome. As Fairbairn's above quote illustrates, as result of her internalisation of relationships to bad objects, the child ends up feeling guilty on one level but *bad to the bone* underneath that. This elucidates the way in which drive theory has the potential to overlook the devastating impact of traumatic abuse and why a model of unconscious phantasy which takes veridical experience into account is essential, as set out in Chapter 3. The relational 'badness' that the child is forced to internalise as a result of abuse therefore equates in extreme cases to 'soul murder':

> Soul murder is my dramatic designation for a certain category of traumatic experiences – those instances of repetitive and chronic overstimulation alternating with emotional deprivation that are deliberately brought about by another individual.
>
> (Shengold, 1979, p. 533)

For Fairbairn, therefore, a central goal of psychotherapy is not only the amelioration of guilt but to 'release' bad objects by orientating clients to benign, good-enough relationships in the outside world. It is essential, then, that the psychotherapist becomes a 'good object' to the client (Fairbairn, 1943, p. 69). I shall consider this 'release of bad objects' later in this chapter and its potentially problematic nature clinically.

Fairbairn acknowledged his early debt to Melanie Klein, and both influenced one another clinically (Mitchell, 1981). However, it is important to note that Fairbairn's use of the term 'bad objects' is distinct from Klein's. For Klein, bad objects are primarily phylogenetic and universal, born of the death instinct and unconscious phantasy, yet for Fairbairn, they are primarily based on libidinal relationships to caregivers: unconscious phantasy is secondary and pathological (Mitchell, 1981). Bad objects do not relate to the death instinct for Fairbairn but are, instead, sequelae from repeated experiences of feeling unlovable and that one's love will always be rejected in the end:

> the greatest need of a child is to obtain conclusive assurance (a) that he is genuinely loved *as a person* by his parents, and (b) that his parents genuinely accept his love.
>
> (Fairbairn, 1941, p. 39; italics my own)

As a result of repeated experiences of emotional abandonment, the child therefore must resort to creating a system of defence against the overwhelming affects of what has now become a relational trauma. Fairbairn therefore postulates that, as a means of coping with the utter devastation of the rejection of her love and her need to be loved, the child internalises these experiences as 'bad objects', which takes place in two stages.[1] In the first stage, the child renders herself 'unconditionally bad' so that those who are tasked with her care may remain 'good', concluding: 'I must be a bad person if they do not love me or want my love' (Fairbairn, 1943). The unconditional badness of this first stage of internalisation is also central to the curse position in terms of forming the sense of immanent lack of belonging/*weirdness*, which contributes to a fated *wyrdness* – to remain repetitively cursed throughout life with no sign of escape. This is the primary curse: the first process of doomed internalisation. This is also richly evocative of the infuriating injustice of the fall and the Calvinist/Puritanical notion of the child being born as a sinner with no say in the matter, cursed from birth to spend the rest of one's life trying to prove otherwise, seeking *redemption*.

Fairbairn states that the abject claustrophobia of becoming a 'sinner' with no possibility of redemption is so unbearable to the child that she then internalises the parts of the caregiver which she considers to be 'good', which sets up a secondary conditional sorcery[2]: 'If only I behave in the way they want, then I will be accepted'. This secondary stage of internalisation is what Fairbairn called the 'moral defence', and it is one of his most poignant contributions in terms of communicating the tragedy of the child becoming a self-appointed carrier of the 'burden of badness' to preserve an omnipotent phantasy, that in cultivating a mysterious and saintly 'goodness' – being a child of God, rather than of Satan – she will be accepted by the rejecting caregiver (Fairbairn, 1943, p. 64). Fairbairn so poignantly illustrates the pact that the child makes with the bad object in the following passage. Although this is often quoted elsewhere, it is too evocative and important not to include here:

> It is better to be a sinner in a world ruled by God than to live in a world ruled by the Devil. A sinner in a world ruled by God may be bad; but there is always a certain sense of security to be derived from the fact that the world around is good – 'God's in His heaven – All's right with the world!'; and in any case there is always a hope of redemption. In a world ruled by the Devil the individual may escape the badness of being a sinner; but he is bad because the world around him is bad. Further, he can have no sense of security and no hope of redemption. The only prospect is one of death and destruction.
>
> (Fairbairn, 1943, pp. 65–66)

The moral defence, then, is that the child exchanges unconditional and libidinal badness for moral and conditional badness. In Fairbairn's paradigm, it is through the conditionality of the moral defence that the superego is established along with its concomitant guilt. Guilt is therefore used as a means of defending against the underlying feelings of shame of needing a bad object to survive 'death and destruction' (1944, p. 93).

I have found Fairbairn's developmental ideas highly instructive in my clinical work and in my development of the curse position, with particular regard to the topography of the primary and secondary curse. As we have seen in previous chapters, the primary curse consists of unconscious phantasies associated with relational trauma and the archaic unconscious. It is at this primary level of the curse position that the individual experiences a particularly ontological shame that she is *faulty*, or 'unconditional badness' in Fairbairn's terms. This immanent shame fosters feelings of alienation, causing the subject to feel that she is toxic to other people. In order to protect against this central core of faultiness, the superego – moral defence – is mobilised to show how the person is *at fault*, which is preferable to feeling *faulty*. The harsh superego of the curse position therefore generates feelings of expecting to be at fault – caught out. This is the classic guilty conscience. These ideas on superego are developed further in the next chapter.

The Case of Christoph Haitzmann

As we have now seen, the moral defence is a renunciative pact between the child's ego and the bad object. Such a pact is commonly found in encounter narratives of familiar spirits in folklore, perhaps most well known in the myth of *Faust*, where a demonic 'familiar' spirit appears and offers magical assistance in exchange for the renunciation of the human soul (Wilby, 2005).

In his 1943 paper concerning the moral defence, Fairbairn examines the pact with regard to Freud's 1922 paper *A Seventeenth-Century Demonological Neurosis*, concerning an impoverished and depressed 17th century artist, Christoph Haitzmann. The Devil appears to Haitzmann at a distressing time in his life when he is incapacitated and unable to work. However, instead of the Faustian offer of untold wealth in exchange for his soul, the bond in this case decrees that the Devil will cure Haitzmann of his melancholy state by 'becoming' his father for nine years. The Devil initially appears to the artist as a kindly male figure but becomes increasingly frightening as he develops the physical attributes with which the Devil is popularly associated – wings and cloven hooves – which, for Freud, betray the first signs of Haitzmann's *ambivalent* feelings towards his father, which also 'governs the relation of mankind to its deity' (Freud, 1923 p. 85). However, as we have seen from the examples in Chapter 1, ambivalence is unbearable to the child and to monotheistic religion. Following Fairbairn's paradigm, it is therefore this ambivalence which leads to the splitting of the object.

Fairbairn chooses to use this part of his 1943 paper as a vehicle for a further critique on Freud's emphasis on the pleasure principle as the determining factor in Haitzmann's psychopathology. This appears to be an oversimplification on Fairbairn's part, as Freud also highlights Haitzmann's ambivalent attachment to his father and his need for security along with his desire for enjoyment. Freud's compassion towards Haitzmann's defensive use of narcissistic phantasies of pleasure is also evident, which he argues are surely preferable to the horrific delusions of punishment which the painter experiences upon entering a holy order to 'cure' himself of his earlier pact. Fairbairn instead contends that it is only by making a pact with God that Haitzmann is cured of his symptoms, which is therefore proof of his theory of a universal need for a good object. Here, Fairbairn seems to discount – or at least skirts over – the ambivalence that Freud specifies, stating only that Haitzmann's admission to the holy order is a 'triumph for the moral defence', which is true in the sense that Haitzmann has become conditionally bad and is now at the mercy of the guilt of the superego (1943, p. 70). Yet there are several other important factors of note. Firstly, Haitzmann's 'cure' comes at the price of a life of masochistic asceticism which can only be considered sadistic on the part of the deity if the only way to be cured of sin is to renounce enjoyment altogether. Secondly, in citing God as the symbol of the 'good object', Fairbairn – perhaps under the influence of his Christian beliefs – ignores the crucial ambivalence that Freud specifies, which is surely one of the key tenets of psychoanalysis. Neither a pact with the Devil or God would have 'saved' Christoph. Perhaps he would have found some peace in accepting his own need for love *and* enjoyment alongside his hostile feelings towards his father. However, I would argue that it is the sadistically wielded carrot of 'good' redemption that is as much, if not more of, a bad object than the Devil himself for Haitzmann. I would therefore agree with Fairbairn's position that it is the primary internalisation of badness which is the most intractable, yet I would argue that this and the moral defence may be compounded by his standpoint of therapist qua redeeming exorcist:

> it may be said of all psychoneurotic and psychotic patients that, if a True Mass is being celebrated in the chancel, a Black Mass is being celebrated in the crypt. It becomes evident, accordingly, that the psychotherapist is the true successor to the exorcist, and that he is concerned, not only with 'the forgiveness of sins', but also with 'the casting out of devils'.
>
> (1943, p. 68)

Fairbairn's metaphors are undeniably evocative and compelling, and there is no doubt that there are similarities between psychotherapy and exorcism in the sense that 'devils' are brought out of the unconscious into the light. However, I find this also sets up a potentially troubling precedent: even if the intention to 'release bad objects' is benign, who are we as therapists to 'know' what must be 'exorcised'? Simply, we are not priests. This may also perpetuate a phantasy that the therapist can 'cure' his clients of all their bad objects – a saviour who will turn inner worlds from the *Dracula* castle into *The Sound of Music*. Fairbairn's notions of redemption from this perspective veer rather too close to demonology at times. It is ironic, then, that with regard to the case of Haitzmann, it is Freud who states that what the artist needed most of all was security. Moreover, this was a security which would have benefitted from being safely ringfenced from any thoughts of redemption.

Endopsychic Structure

In 1944's *Endopsychic Structure Considered in Terms of Object-Relationships*, Fairbairn develops an 'anatomic scaffolding for the unconscious' which maintains his repudiation of an epistemology of the drives and continues his absolute focus on the libidinal attachment to internal and external objects (Grotstein, 2014, p. xxi).

As a result of the child's intolerable frustration of emotional experience, the child splits the aspect of the caregiver identified with this traumatic rejection – the bad object – into two: the rejecting and exciting object (Fairbairn, 1944; Ogden, 2010). Fairbairn postulates that there is a part of the child's ego which is libidinally attached to the rejecting object and the other to the exciting object (Fairbairn, 1944; Ogden, 2010). As a result of its aggression towards these dependent parts of the ego, the 'central ego' therefore splits off *these newly formed ego object dyads* and represses them (Ogden, 2010). This effectively constitutes a secondary repression of bad objects to that described in the 1943 paper with the moral defence.[3] The 'libidinal' ('people-pleasing') ego craves love from the 'exciting' (alluring, seductive) part object identified with the caregiver and the resentfully wounded 'anti-libidinal ego' is tied to a rejecting, abandoning part object identified with the caregiver (Ogden, 2010). These bi-lateral split-off dyads are locked in a masochistic oscillation between longing for acceptance and feeling resentment.

It is important to note – particularly from a clinical perspective – that a further stage of repression also takes place in Fairbairn's endopsychic structure. The hostility of the anti-libidinal/rejecting object cathexis also extends to attempting to emotionally annihilate the 'needy' libidinal self which is repeatedly tantalised by the exciting object but never has its needs met. The security and loving tenderness which the libidinal ego craves is sabotaged by the anti-libidinal ego, which associates any feelings of vulnerability with rejection and shame. This is why Fairbairn also refers to the anti-libidinal ego as the 'internal saboteur' (1944). The internal saboteur, therefore, exists as a means of protection from the original devastating traumatic experiences. The constant self-attacks on one's need for love are therefore a small price to pay, as they protect the individual from the primary curse of a harrowing form of shame which Fairbairn heartrendingly describes as 'beggardom'.

> At a somewhat deeper level (or at an earlier stage) the experience is one of shame over the display of needs which are disregarded or belittled. In virtue of these experiences of humiliation and shame he feels reduced to a state of worthlessness, destitution or beggardom.
>
> (Fairbairn, 1944, p. 113)

Clinically, therefore, it is well worth considering how much aggression is *intra-psychically cathected* at the expense of protecting others from the hurt and dependent aspects of the self. Aggression is felt to be particularly perilous, as it is perceived as being so closely linked with abandonment. This again is driven by an implicit conditionality of the moral defence – 'If I protect others from my neediness and aggression, then they won't reject me' – and is also an effort to remedy the primary curse of libidinal faultiness: the anti-libidinal ego *hates* libidinal attachments due to the implicit dread of rejection – almost as much as the shame of being witnessed in one's neediness. It therefore presents a double bind for such clients: one has to deal with either the shame of being witnessed in her need or the toxic effects of holding on to excruciating aggression and loneliness. I believe this to be an extraordinary contribution from Fairbairn, as this theory, accompanied by the moral defence, provides the most plausible explanations I have come across for a particularly masochistic form of relational repetition compulsion from which the individual cannot escape.

The People Pleaser/Saviour/Empath/Narcissist

Clients who suffer relational trauma of this nature will tend to choose partners with whom they can play out the agonising *jouissance* of oscillating between excitement and rejection, and this is relevant for clients who refer to themselves as 'people pleasers' or 'saviours'. The people pleaser/saviour sincerely believes that she wants to save others yet is participating in a painful drama where the person she wishes to 'save' has been unconsciously selected so that they may fulfil a phantasy that the original trauma can be reversed and that her love will be accepted (on the condition that she behaves accordingly – that she is 'good'). Of course, as she is re-enacting her developmental trauma – which often involves abuse and/or neglect – being 'good' can tragically often mean expecting and perhaps even seeking out abusive experiences and relationships.

As the object relations take place within what Fairbairn calls a 'closed system', it seems to the individual that she wishes to save or please others in a particularly virtuous way, but she is only responding libidinally to the demands of bad objects and therefore stuck in a masochistic loop (Fairbairn, 1994). She desperately would love to save herself but is imprisoned by her pathological object relations. It is important to therefore note that the supposed self-sacrifice of wanting to 'save' or 'please' others also conforms to the narrative of trying to become 'good' and thereby gaining the caregiver's (bad object's) love and becoming loveable, which also keeps the person in the position of the conditionally bad victim. In this scenario, the individual selects partners to whom they quickly develop a rejecting or exciting transference which they can oscillate between and who are often now popularly described as having a 'narcissistic' personality. There are countless online videos and blogs about 'empaths' and 'narcissists' and advice for what empaths can do to stop getting hurt. My perspective on this is that the creation of these toxic couplings is effectively a form of re-enactment of the original trauma. The 'empath' identifies with the (narcissistic) bad objects (rejecting/exciting) and wishes the chosen person to accept her love so that she then no longer feels unconditionally bad. This then results in a paradox because, in the mind of the 'empath', she needs to prove that she is 'good' by 'saving' the 'narcissist' from being bad. In spite of this, at a libidinal level, this is the last thing she wants, as she is lost in a closed system of identifying with one or another ego-bad object coupling: if the narcissist one day suddenly starts showing signs of being an 'empath', he/she will be rejected right away, as her anti-libidinal ego will associate him/her with her neediness. This may go some way to explain why traumatised people choose abusive partners.

Case Illustration: 'Home Truths'

Ms. A., a woman in her late 20s, had been attending weekly therapy for almost a year. She was the youngest of three, with two older brothers. Ms. A.'s parents had both had a strict religious upbringing, and the family attended mass every Sunday. Ms. A. described family dinners as a 'recurring nightmare', as her parents always insisted that they all sit down to dinner 'as a family', and the stilted conversations that ensued often had 'an undertow'. She always felt she needed to be hypervigilant around her mother, who would sometimes fly into a rage for what Ms. A. saw as apparently trivial motives. Ms. A. remembers spilling her soup down her jumper when she was 12, and her mother cruelly reprimanded her and called her 'a clumsy moron'. Ms. A. recalls that her father 'just sat there', but her eldest brother had stood up for her and told her mother that she had been 'out of order'. Sadly for Ms. A., her eldest brother left home when she was 14, and the other brother left shortly after, which left her to deal with her parents' frequent rows, which would sometimes escalate into physical violence. Ms. A. recalls sometimes consoling her mother after these arguments, and it had been a way for them to become 'closer'. However, her mother usually had been drinking on these occasions, and despite Ms. A. feeling that she had helped her mother feel better, her mother would always use this as an occasion – under the guise of caring maternal advice – to criticise her and to tell her 'home truths'. Despite her mother's protestations otherwise, Ms. A. always felt as if she was being told that she needed to change who she was, not only what she did. This same dynamic continued to the present day, as whenever she called her mother for reassurance about her boyfriend or work, when she came off the call, she tended to feel that there was something wrong with her and that this was the reason why these problems would arise.

In today's session, after several minutes of talking about how under pressure she felt at work – where she worked many more hours than she was paid for – Ms. A. said that she was 'sick and tired' of her relationship with her boyfriend. Ms. A. had called him six times the night before and still had not heard from him. She had also messaged him several times and received notifications that he had seen the messages. When I suggested that this must be difficult for her not to have heard back from him, she looked back with a mixture of puzzlement and disdain. She said that she didn't see how it was any more difficult for her than anybody else and that she felt like a 'pathetic idiot' for being so 'clingy'. I suddenly felt wounded and a burning, pinching sensation in my solar plexus as if I had been emotionally stabbed. I became conscious that my cheeks felt like they were burning and that I, too, was not only *pathetic* but also insincere due to what I now felt was a rather pat intervention. In saying, 'That must be really difficult for you', I had somehow unwittingly placed myself on a condescending pedestal, where the implicit message was 'to be so clingy and never become like me, who is not bothered by such things'. To use Fairbairn's metaphors, I was now the priest up there in the chancel, and this had been Ms. A.'s way of pulling me down to the black mass.

After several moments of silence, which felt charged with a precarious sense of expectation, I asked Ms. A. if we could think together about what had just happened. Although she retained her look of puzzlement, I then asked her what it had been like for her when I had said, 'It must have been difficult for you'. Ms. A. replied that she hadn't really thought much about it and as she looked at me, I now saw a helplessness in her eyes. I also felt helpless and that I was now, instead, slowly falling into the crypt of shame as 'Here I am, making it about me' by asking Ms. A. to think about the transference. I felt like I was being punished for something, but wasn't sure by whom exactly, or for what.

Shortly afterwards, I experienced a 'meta-awareness' where I could somehow observe myself thinking, 'I might take another stab at what this might be about', almost as if someone else were saying it in my mind – perhaps a 'changeling' therapist, but not me. I then became acutely aware of the uncanny nature of this countertransference – especially the disturbing potency of the word 'stab' – and again felt a flush of shame, as if, even though I had not said it out loud, I had colluded with some hostile internal object in the field that was now firmly in control.

After a few more moments and managing to compose myself a little more, I said – now as 'myself' again, feeling that I could now perhaps see a way out of the crypt – 'I'd like to explore this with you but also can't help noticing that I might get it wrong, or what I say might be hard for you to hear'. Ms. A. looked somewhat baffled and scared at the same time, as if it were now I that was going to 'stab' her in revenge by telling her something that I thought she 'needed' to hear. At this moment I could not put this feeling into words in my mind, but it felt like something hostile that could not be contained and had to be evacuated. I therefore decided it was best to say nothing further at this point. Ms. A. then asked me with a smile that appeared once again, uncannily dislocated from her words – 'Well, is there something you think I need to know? Because if you do, it's better that you tell me – it's why I come here after all'. I felt entirely flummoxed by this statement, as it had not gone the way I had expected (though I don't think I knew what I expected). I then began to feel like I was now being saved from being sacrificed in the black mass by inflation and was floating back up to the godliness of the chancel – the priest who would impart pious wisdom to his client from the pulpit. I felt an immense pressure at this moment. I wanted to respond compassionately, yet I was conscious that I did not wish to respond with the solemn grandiosity that I felt Ms. A. expected. I therefore said, 'I feel as if I am now expected to tell you a "home truth", though I don't actually have one I can think of at this moment'. I now felt pathetic and helpless again, which troubled me, but at least I was now a *human* again, and I sensed from Ms. A.'s reaction that she saw this helplessness in me. Ms. A. laughed, and I felt that, in my floundering on my way back up to the 'chancel', she felt compassion for me, and this laugh had finally popped this persecutory intersubjective bubble somehow and had brought us both back to the consulting room. I had now become a flawed human being again who happened to be her therapist rather than a malevolent satanist or a wise, virtuous priest.

After a short pause, Ms. A. seemed to grow in confidence and said to me, smiling once more, though now in a more relaxed, even playful way, 'You know, I've always hated the phrase "home truths", as it's super depressing'. I asked her why she thought so. 'Well, I guess that there's something in it that suggests that other people know what's best for you, when they really don't!' Ms. A.'s eyes then suddenly filled with tears, and she quickly looked down at the floor and then straight at me before fully bursting into tears: 'And I'm sick of doing this to myself'. She then said that she wished that she could end the relationship with her boyfriend but couldn't do it, and maybe this was the 'home truth' she had been choosing to ignore.

After some moments, I said that it felt to me as if there was somehow something more about the phrase 'home truths' that we hadn't thought about but still seemed important. Then suddenly, feeling a rush of enthused adrenaline I said: 'Now I'm fairly sure you told me in the first session that "home truths" was a phrase your mother used to use'. At this, Ms. A. smiled again and said drily, 'Yes, I know, I was wondering whether you'd remember'. There were now some moments of silence where Ms. A. appeared to be lost deep in thought. Curiously, Ms. A. then told me that she hadn't realised that she knew that she had been waiting for me to make the link until I had said it aloud.

Discussion

We can see from this case illustration how the initial 'pat' intervention, though intended to ease Ms. A.'s internal saboteur, had unconsciously set myself up as an ego-ideal therapist, which was received as a reminder of the futile impossibility of the 'moral defence' at a time when Ms. A. was desperately attempting to be loved by and have her love accepted by a boyfriend who she felt rejected by and punished by through his silence. Her harsh self-criticism had been an attack on her libidinal ego by its anti-libidinal counterpart. My 'supportive and empathic' intervention only spoke to Ms. A.'s hurt anti-libidinal ego, which she experienced as condescending to her libidinal ego, which the anti-libidinal ego despised and perceived as 'pathetic'. As the split ego dynamics take place at an unconscious level, the verbal attack was thus perceived consciously to be on herself, yet I also experienced the emotional 'knife' counter-transferentially. The atmosphere of imminent attack was potent in this session, evoking family dinner dynamics, where this emotional blade used threat and shame to sever the possibility that emotions can be thought about rather than acted upon. These powerful threats of being emotionally stabbed relate to the burning sensation in the solar plexus I experienced, and it was Ms. A.'s anti-libidinal ego which wielded the knife.

It is important to note that as I was on my way home from the session, I continued to reflect on my 'pat' intervention and its sense of insincerity which still bothered me somehow: I was now alone with my own anti-libidinal ego. Indeed, I thought to myself, it could be considered insincere in the sense that my 'pat' intervention perhaps had been rather generic and unimaginative, yet I felt curious about the harshness of my superego and a jarring affective ambivalence I felt following Ms. A.'s response to the intervention. I had felt pathetic *and* insincere at the same time; a clingy(ing), need(iness) to find the right words, which so uncomfortably folded into a feeling of narcissistic artifice and superiority; and a bizarre sense of *alien mutuality*. I considered that this could have been the result of my identification with the exciting object and the libidinal ego which had been projected into me. As the identification took hold, it seemed that everything I thought and felt represented an aggressive retaliation of the 'home truths': I had become Ms. A.'s mother. These phantasies were so powerful at this point that I felt almost as if Ms. A. would *hear my thought* – perhaps a re-enactment of the traumatic clairvoyance between her and her mother and Ms. A.'s need to disown her own aggression for fear of retaliation and abandonment. This disavowal of anti-libidinal rage – not wishing to carry the 'burden of badness' – could also account for the uncanny dissociative doubling of the 'phantom therapist' in the countertransference: my own experience of the desire to split off violent thoughts associated with rejection.

These violent feelings that were projected in the transference appeared to represent an important enactment. Ms. A. had projected the persecutory feelings of feeling 'pathetic' and 'clingy' into me to see how *I* would deal with them. When Ms. A. asked me to tell her 'what she needs to know', I was invited to become another authority figure who would impose 'home truths' upon her, yet instead of retaliating as a rejecting mother object, I involuntarily conveyed my inherent powerlessness to do so, which Ms. A. could now see was not 'pathetic' but simply human. In witnessing my fallibility and 'neediness' to be seen as making the 'right' intervention, Ms. A. could experience compassion for me in the transference, which she could then internalise for herself, thereby reducing the harshness of her attacks by her anti-libidinal ego on its libidinal counterpart, which Fairbairn highlights as the second aim of psychoanalytic treatment (Fairbairn, 1994, p. 182).

It is important to note that Ms. A. didn't realise that she had been waiting for me to make the link between the phrase and internal mother object until I said it aloud, and this therefore indicated an intersubjective *telepathic expectation*: she had unconsciously been waiting for me to make the link, and I had unconsciously known she had been expecting it. Ms. A.'s awareness that she had already – if unconsciously – made the link between the use of the phrase 'home truths' and the internal bad (mother) object therefore became pivotal in terms of facilitating an embodied feeling of agency in the therapeutic relationship. This met one of the principal treatment aims identified by Fairbairn, as Ms. A. was able to utilise the therapeutic relationship as a means of exchanging 'infantile dependency' for adult agency (Fairbairn, 1994, p. 182). Indeed, Fairbairn postulates that it is the therapeutic relationship *at both a transference and person-to-person level* which heals the pathological libidinal attachments to bad objects (Fairbairn, 1994). In this case illustration, at the 'moment of meeting' where Ms. A. and I each realised the link between the phrase and the bad object, we then moved from a transference to a person-to-person relationship (Stern et al., 1998). This also illustrates the importance of both forms of relationship in terms of treating relational trauma.

Concluding Comments

Despite the imperfections which are set out in this chapter, Fairbairn offers us an 'object relations theory of the personality' which provides us with an invaluable resource for deciphering the role of relational trauma and its powerful influence on the intractability and repetition compulsion of the curse position. For Fairbairn, the overarching factor in treating relational trauma and 'breaching' the closed system of the curse is the development of a therapeutic relationship (1994, p. 174). Fairbairn's work has therefore become an important blueprint for relational approaches to heal what I call the primary curse. Despite having the benefit of Fairbairn's work as a resource, it can be challenging to work with clients who cannot seem to exit from the pathological relationships in which they find themselves and which can cause anxiety in the therapist. In my own experience, I have found it can therefore be hard to resist the temptation to 'reason' with clients about whether abusive relationships are 'good' for them. Of course, they know full well they are not. This only results in the client closing off as the therapist is perceived as a threat to maintaining the relationship with bad objects to which they have become addicted or the therapist is experienced as a superego figure who 'knows' what's best. It is important therefore to work in the transference to become an object which is thoughtful yet fallible and human. Through working in this way and by helping clients to make links between their internal object worlds and their repetition compulsions in the outer world, they therefore have an opportunity to begin to populate their inner world with objects that represent attachment security as opposed to painful dependence.

Notes

1 In his earlier papers, Fairbairn focuses on the oral introjection of objects, which is now replaced by internalising. See Mitchell (1981).
2 I refer to Frazer's definition of sorcery: 'Do this so that this may happen' (Frazer and Fraser, 1994, p. 33).
3 'The "central ego" is a dynamic structure, from which . . . the other mental structures are subsequently derived' (Fairbairn, 1944, p. 106).

References

Fairbairn, R. (1941 [1952]). A Revised Psychopathology of the Psychoses and Psychoneuroses. In W. R. Fairbairn, *Psychoanalytic Studies of the Personality*. London: Routledge and Kegan Paul.

Fairbairn, R. (1943 [1952]). The Repression and the Return of Bad Objects (with Special Reference to the War Neuroses). In W. R. Fairbairn, *Psychoanalytic Studies of the Personality*. London: Routledge and Kegan Paul.

Fairbairn, R. (1994). On the Nature and Aims of Psychoanalytical Treatment. In W. R. D. Scharff and E. F. Birtles (eds), *From Instinct to Self: Selected Papers of W.R.D. Fairbairn* (J. Aronson). www.freepsychotherapybooks.org. Accessed 28/09/2022.

Fairbairn, W. R. D. (1944 [1952]). Endopsychic Structure Considered in Terms of Object-Relationships. In W. R. Fairbairn, *Psychoanalytic Studies of the Personality*. London: Routledge and Kegan Paul.

Frazer, J. and Fraser, R. (1994). *The Golden Bough*. Oxford: Oxford University Press.

Freud, S. (1923 [1922]). A Seventeenth-Century Demonological Neurosis. In J. Strachey (ed), *The Standard Edition of the Complete Psychological Works of Sigmund Freud, Volume XIX (1923–1925): The Ego and the Id and Other Works*. London: The Hogarth Press and the Institute of Psychoanalysis, pp. 1–308.

Grotstein, J. (2014). Introduction. In D. E. Scharff and G. S. Clarke (eds), *Fairbairn and the Object Relations Tradition*. London: Karnac Books, pp. xxi–xxii.

Hoffman, M. T. and Hoffmann, L. W. (2014). Religion in the Life and Work of W. R. D. Fairbairn. In S. C. Clarke and D. E. Scharff (eds), *Fairbairn and the Object Relations Tradition*. London: Karnac.

Mitchell, S. (1981). The origin and nature of the "object" in the theories of Klein and Fairbairn. *Contemporary Psychoanalysis*, 17(3): 374–398.

Ogden, T. H. (1983). The concept of internal object relations. *The International Journal of Psychoanalysis*, 64(2): 227–241.

Ogden, T. H. (2010). Why read Fairbairn? *The International Journal of Psychoanalysis*, 91(1): 101–118.

Shengold, L. L. (1979). Child abuse and deprivation: Soul murder. *Journal of the American Psychoanalytic Association*, 27(3): 533–559.

Sinason, V. (2014). Fairbairn: Abuse, Trauma, and Multiplicity. In D. E. Scharff and G. S. Clarke (eds), *Fairbairn and the Object Relations Tradition*. London: Karnac Books, pp. 197–208.

Stern, D. N., Sander, L. W et al. (1998). Non-interpretative mechanisms in psychoanalytic therapy: The "something more" than interpretation. *International Journal of Psycho-Analysis*, 79: 903–921.

Wilby, E. (2005). *Cunning Folk and Familiar Spirits: Shamanistic Visionary Tradition in Early Modern British Witchcraft and Magic*. Brighton: Sussex Academic Press.

Chapter 8

The Devil's Culpa
Shame, Guilt, & Evil

Introduction

This chapter continues along the line of the previous chapter's affective themes of shame and guilt, though with a particular focus on the way in which these affects individually and interdependently contribute to the curse position, through the shame of the ideal-ego and the persecutory guilt of the superego. The alienating narcissistic shame of the ideal-ego is then illustrated through the doomed imaginary of Lacan's *mirror stage* and its intersubjective corollaries.

The immanent 'badness' of the subject in the curse position and the unconscious sense of guilt and need for punishment can be experienced as, and conflated with, *being evil*, resulting in what I call *culpevility*. As the repressive aspects of the ego-ideal and the superego are antithetical to one another's aims, this can create profound conflicts, particularly within the traumatised subject. These vicissitudes are illustrated through David Lindsay's *A Voyage to Arcturus*, David Lynch's *Lost Highway*, and a case illustration.

The Ego-ideal and the Superego

As we have seen from the previous chapter, there is an interdependence between two forms of 'badness' in the curse position: the inherent 'faultiness' of the primary curse and the guilt-based defences of its secondary counterpart.

In this chapter, I set out to build on these ideas by looking into further contributory elements of superego functioning, guilt, and – through the 'ego-ideal' – shame (Freud, 1914).

It is important to note that although Freud often used the terms ego-ideal and superego interchangeably, in the interests of clarity, I find it most useful to maintain the specified distinction.[1]

According to Freud, the 'ego-ideal' stems from primary narcissism, a stage of 'new psychical action', where the ego itself becomes the object of libido (Freud, 1914; Kanzer, 1964). Primary narcissism was originally postulated by Freud as a result of the analysis of patients with schizophrenia, where object libido was seen to be significantly depleted, resulting in a secondary form of narcissism which

DOI: 10.4324/9781003168027-9

manifests in megalomania (Freud, ibid.). Freud therefore posits that this secondary narcissism sits topographically upon the 'original libidinal cathexis of the ego' or 'primary narcissism', a 'magical' stage of being in love with oneself (ibid.). During the primary stage of narcissism, the subject perceives objects as extensions of oneself, and object libido is therefore entirely absent. However, as we have seen through the developmental research cited in Chapter 3, the world of the infant is an interpersonal one, where proto expectations based on internal representations of mutual interactions are present as early as the first few months of life. For Beebe and Lachmann, these therefore become the basis of one's expectations and ideals:

> Our basic proposal is that early interaction structures provide an important basis for the organization of infant experience and emerging self- and object representations. Interaction structures are characteristic patterns of mutual regulations in which both infant and caretaker influence each other. The infant comes to recognize, remember, and *expect* these recurring interaction structures.
>
> (Beebe and Lachmann, 1988, p. 306; italics my own)

Yet for Freud, despite the mirage of mutuality, parental love and falling in love are driven by narcissistic libido:

> Parental love, which is so moving and at bottom so childish, is nothing but the parents' narcissism born again, which, transformed into object-love, unmistakably reveals its former nature.
>
> (Freud, 1914, p. 91)

The way in which parental love is bound up with narcissism and its related failed projects suggests a precarious prospect for the infant if, as Freud suggests, this leads to idealistic projections onto – as Freud puts it – 'his majesty the baby'.

> . . . he shall not be subject to the necessities which they have recognized as paramount in life. Illness, death, renunciation of enjoyment, restrictions on his own will, shall not touch him; the laws of nature and of society shall be abrogated in his favour; he shall once more really be the centre and core of creation – 'His Majesty the Baby', as we once fancied ourselves.
>
> (Freud, 1914, p. 91)

For Winnicott, it is instead the 'holding environment' provided by the mother which determines the expectations and ideals of the child and the overarching factor in terms of translating potential into its realisation (1960, p. 589). This developmental realisation, of course, will depend on the caregiver's own 'empathy and awareness' – not normally traits associated with narcissism – and the extent to which one can accept the renunciation of one's own will and enjoyment and one's baby's (ibid.). However, in cases where there are significant deficits in empathy, there is also a danger that the potential of the child can become bound up with the (ego-ideal) expectations of the caregiver who cannot think of the infant as a separate object, which the infant will inevitably introject.

Freud's ego-ideal, then, is constructed out of a narcissistic ideal: it is about 'how we fancy ourselves', and how we see our children will be defined in these terms. Freud asserts that the ego-ideal is the 'conditioning factor of repression', and what the ego deems will be unacceptable to this benchmarking agency must therefore be defended against (Freud, 1914, p. 94). This narcissistic, omnipotent projection forms the basis of our ideals and ambitions later in life.

> This ideal ego is now the target of the self-love which was enjoyed in childhood by the actual ego. The subject's narcissism makes its appearance displaced on to this new ideal ego, which, like the infantile ego, finds itself possessed of every perfection that is of value. As always where the libido is concerned, man has here again shown himself incapable of giving up a satisfaction he had once enjoyed. He is not willing to forgo the narcissistic perfection of his childhood; and when, as he grows up, he is disturbed by the admonitions of others and by the awakening of his own critical judgement, so that he can no longer retain that perfection, he seeks to recover it in the new form of an ego ideal. What he projects before him as his ideal is the substitute for the lost narcissism of his childhood in which he was his own ideal.
>
> (ibid.)

The Narcissistic Eye

The ego-ideal, then, is narcissistically invested in, and in cases where too much libido is cathected to the ego, perceiving oneself to have fallen short can become a profound source of shame. These ideals are constructed through interactions with caregivers along with their associated expectations, desires, and identifications.

> It would not surprise us if we were to find a special psychical agency which performs the task of seeing that narcissistic satisfaction from the ego-ideal is ensured and which, with this end in view, constantly watches the actual ego and measures it by that ideal.
>
> (Freud, 1914, p. 95)

Based on Freud's perspective here, we can consider the ego-ideal to be one aspect of the superego, a 'narcissistic eye' – akin to Freud's 'purified pleasure ego' (1915, p. 135). Based on Beebe and Lachmann's research, I would argue that this 'narcissistic eye' consists of myriad representations[2] of endogenous and external interactions. As the infant matures, the corollary of this process becomes an increasing awareness of the existence of one's ego-ideal: as a result of the narcissistic eye's roots in identification, one becomes increasingly aware of its *outsideness*.

Freud suggests that it is this perception of externality which leads to phantasies of being observed (1973 [1917], p. 479).

When the infant reaches the Oedipal stage of parental prohibition, the narcissistic eye and its concomitant wounds become embedded within a secondary ocular framework of the law: this is where shame meets guilt. The wordless shame internalised from the pre-Oedipal stage now combines with the 'unconscious sense of guilt/need for punishment' associated with the superego/conscience (Freud, 1961 [1923]). I would argue therefore that much of the shame that is associated with the ego-ideal stems from the earliest stage of mental functioning and accounts for the intractability of the primary curse (Fairbairn, 1943). Heinz Kohut highlights the primitive and non-adaptive element of narcissistic libido: as one develops, this irresistible force becomes a profound source of shame, which

> arises when the ego is unable to provide a proper discharge for the exhibitionistic demands of the narcissistic self.
>
> (Kohut, 1966, p. 244)

Given the uncompromising nature of narcissistic libido, the blocking function of shame or the prohibitions of guilt work against fulfilling the desire of the subject. This helps to account for why narcissistic presentations are particularly challenging in clinical settings.

We can now see the way in which two functions of superego work in opposition to one another and are antithetical to the ego: the narcissistic eye represses all that does not meet the image of an ideal self, yet such repressions will often not match those which are conducted by the superego. The ego therefore must not only contend with conflict between itself and 'three tyrannical masters',[3] but also between the ego-ideal and the superego. Freud illustrates this struggle in *Civilisation and Its Discontents*:

> To renounce the drives is no longer enough, for the desire persists and cannot be concealed from the superego. Despite one's renunciation, then, a sense of guilt will arise . . . – loss of love, and punishment at the hands of the external authority – has been exchanged for an enduring inner unhappiness, the tension created by the consciousness of guilt.
>
> (2002, p. 82)

The Mirror

Lacan's 'mirror phase' is posited to take place between 6 and 18 months (Lacan, 2006). The child 'recognises' herself in the reflected mirror, yet this is merely an illusory *méconnaissance*, as the 'imago' – what Lacan calls *l'objet petit a* – which she sees is an alluring mirage of wholeness, the tantalising obverse of her ontological fragmentation (ibid.). The child's ego is therefore made up of purely of imaginary identifications. The narcissistic eye which stares out of the mirror creates a psychic hole in the subject, which is then affectively experienced as an eternal grasping 'lack' (Lacan, 2006, p. 807). This lack is the basis of desire – for wanting what one can never have.

Due to the inevitable deficits and disappointments that fall between expectation and actuality, the imaginary world (unconscious phantasy) offers *supplementary gratifications to the nascent expectations of the infant*. In lieu of a containing environment, the child becomes increasingly susceptible to a seductive *méconnaissance* which inevitably leads to subsequent disturbance, as this interferes with symbolic functioning:

> confusions in the symbolic stem from the imaginary – this has been known forever, which is an explanation for aggressive and paranoiac[4] defences.
>
> (Lacan, 2006, p. 607)

Lacan's three dimensions of psychic functioning – the real, imaginary, and symbolic – therefore provide us with a helpful model of reference for the curse position. As a result of the expectations of the imaginary register, subsequent developmental entry into the symbolic realm of language is therefore already compromised in infancy. However, when one is faced with ruptures in symbolisation which are caused by 'the real' (the 'remainder' of trauma which cannot be thought about), one attempts to use the imaginary (the illusion of wholeness) to fill the resultant void, which becomes a compulsion to repeat. These cycles of rupture then themselves become a source of shame, as one can never meet the demands of the narcissistic eye (*l'objet petit a*). The symbolisation of the real is also antithetical to the preservation of the imaginary (which the subject becomes masochistically invested in), thereby ensuring that the curse remains in place. As we saw from the previous chapter, one then becomes a 'people pleaser' as an adult – narcissistically invested in the desire of *l'objet petit a*.

> The mirror phase establishes the framework for intersubjective illusion insofar as it enables the child now to mirror the mother's desire, to be what the mother wants so as to please her.
>
> (Muller, 1985, p. 238)

The desire of the imago mother drives an early yearning in the infant, driven by the identifications of the imaginary. However, if the infant is faced with unpredictable or neglectful caregivers with their own imaginary preoccupations, this

> strains the baby to the limits of his or her capacity to allow for events. This brings a threat of chaos, and the baby will organize withdrawal, or will not look except to perceive, as a defence. A baby so treated will grow up puzzled about mirrors and what the mirror has to offer. If the mother's face is unresponsive, then a mirror is a thing to be looked at but not to be looked into.
>
> (Winnicott, 2005, p. 152)

This 'looking at' rather than 'into' then itself becomes a driver of narcissistic de-fences, where intimacy is avoided as it is perceived as a threat to the self, and an imago supplements an object relationship. We saw such an illustration of this kind of relationship in Chapter 4 between Nathaniel and Olympia in 'The Sandman'. Staying within the phantasy of the imaginary thus offers the subject an illusory life free of vulnerability and rejection.

Guilt and Evil

Aside from the above considerations regarding libidinal badness driven by shame and guilt, I would now like to deepen this analysis by exploring the curious rela-tionship between guilt and evil as psychic defences. A current of this 'badness' runs through guilt and evil, yet when a person who suffers from abuse or neglect by their caregiver(s) then locates the 'evil' within themselves, this points to a particularly pathological form of identification with the aggressor (Ferenczi, 1988). This form of identification is chillingly illustrated in David Lindsay's gnostic sci-fi fantasy *A Voyage to Arcturus*. The story is set on planet Tormance, a part of the Arcturus star system, to which its hero, Maskull, travels on a quest from Earth. Tormance is ruled over by Crystalman, a *demiurgic* deity who seduces his population into worship-ping him through the currency of pleasure. Yet there is a price to pay: each time an inhabitant dies on Tormance, his/her face chillingly transmogrifies into the 'mask' of Crystalman and develops a 'vulgar, sordid bestial grin', indicating a demonic theft of the soul (Lindsay, 1920).

> Crystalman is Blake's Satanic Urizen, or Yeats's Will, the Freudian super-ego or the Jupiter of Prometheus Unbound.
>
> (Bloom, 1982, p. 214)

Crystalman is also reminiscent of the malignant, 'changeling' superego we en-countered in Chapter 6: as a result of developmental trauma, this sadistic *demiurgic* conscience takes the place of the parent by berating the child, telling her that she is bad and evil. The child begins to believe that everything that her innate attachment needs for love and tenderness are 'evil' transgressions which have a destructive ef-fect on others for which she must feel guilty. It is this affective phenomenon which I call *culpevility*: the Devil's culpa. The Devil's culpa is the shadow – demonic – side of the *daimon* which the child introjects and identifies with. This culpevility is redolent of Neumann's 'primal guilt', where the child feels scapegoated as the 'black sheep' who is identified with the demon *Azazel* and brings a particularly 'evil' misfortune upon one's family (in Perera, 1986, p. 15).

> Individuals identified with the scapegoat archetype feel themselves to be the carriers of shamefully evil behaviors and attitudes that disrupt relationships – that discomfort the parental figure. On the magicmatriarchal level, where part stands for whole, they identify with the stuff branded 'wrong' or 'ugly' or

'bad'. The rejection is often enough unconscious, or it is rationalized in super-ego terms (both by the parent and by the scapegoat), but its roots lie deeper. It is not what the child has done that brings rejection, but what the child is in relation to the parent. The child has been found different and thus threatening and hateful.

(Perera, 1986, p. 15)

The 'magic-matriarchal' level which Perera identifies of primal guilt there-fore indicates that it is caused by a combination of the archaic unconscious, unconscious phantasy, and developmental trauma. When the child has inter-nalised badness to this degree of severity, all her ideals become tainted by her culpevility.

Let us consider at this point the way in which the ego-ideal and the hopes and aspirations of the *daimonic* spirit can be affected by the cruelty of the superego. If this trauma is left untreated, it may have catastrophic consequences on one's capac-ity to individuate.

Individuation means becoming an 'in-dividual', and, in so far as 'individual-ity' embraces our innermost, last, and incomparable uniqueness, it also implies becoming one's own self. We could therefore translate individuation as 'coming to selfhood' or 'self-realization'.

(Jung, 1966, p. 238)

Yet aside from trauma, individuation always carries a cost: to 'individuate' from the perspective of the gods is a transgression of their will and therefore results in what Jung calls 'Promethean guilt', a 'taboo infringement' tantamount to the theft of fire (Jung and Hull, 1966, p. 671). The Promethean 'whims of the conscious mind' may lead us to get what we want, yet we become alienated from our commu-nities, symbolically 'chained to the lonely cliffs of the Caucasus, forsaken of God and man' (Jung and Hull, 1966, pp. 671–672).

You came to steal Muspel-fire, to give a deeper life to men – never doubting if your soul could endure burning.

(Lindsay, 1920, p. 194)

Bloom postulates that Maskull – like other Promethean characters such as Frank-enstein and Don Quixote – cannot separate their narcissism from their Promethean-ism (1982, pp. 211–212). It is Maskull's 'never doubting' narcissism which enables Crystalman – who for Bloom represents superego – to deceive him, which leads to his eventual demise. Despite Maskull's conscious Promethean goal, it is his unconscious narcissism which leads him identify with the *demiurge* (Bloom, 1982, p. 219). *In one's Promethean quest for freedom from and to rebel against author-ity, it is our narcissism which can lead us to unconsciously identify with the dark aspects of that same authority.*

These conflicts between Prometheanism and narcissism serve as helpful mythological symbols to think about the difference between pathological narcissistic desire and one's desire to individuate and fulfil one's *daimonic* potential. Jung's and Bloom's mythological insights therefore offer new perspectives into Freud's emphasis on the pathological nature of ego-ideal/ideal-ego, which, as we have seen, Freud uses interchangeably. Hanly sees this as a missed opportunity for Freud, and therefore proposes a separation of the two, noting the *potential* of ego-ideal (daimonic spirit) versus the pathological ideal-ego (1984, p. 253). Indeed, if the 'potential' aspect of ego-ideal is only framed in pathological terms, surely there is a risk that one's legitimate ideals become conflated with the grandiosity of secondary narcissism. In a Western culture where 'narcissism' is commonly levelled as an insult, one may easily start to think one's own desires to find a better job, create art, or feel proud of one's achievements are 'narcissistic'.

In genuine cases of destructive narcissism, it is, of course, undoubtedly essential that the therapist does not collude with his client's defences, yet colluding with the conflation of narcissism and aspiration is also antithetical to psychotherapeutic growth. Moreover, for clients who have experienced significant narcissistic wounding and shame, it is already hard for them to separate benign from narcissistic aspirations. For this client group, therapy therefore becomes an important means of facilitating a compassionate understanding of the difference between the destructive nature of identifying with the narcissistic imaginary and the *daimonic* ideals which propel one's individuation. Importantly, when working with clients who operate from the curse position, the therapist is not only working with the collision between the ego-ideal and the superego (which, Freud highlights, applies to us all) but also the additionally distorting aspect of relational trauma, which results in a cocktail of shame and persecutory guilt. As we have seen, clients who feel scapegoated by their families may come to frame their past actions in terms of their immanent 'evil'. They thus become 'libidinally attached' to guilt and evil as bad objects (Fairbairn, 1943). These bad objects generate what Freud calls a 'sense of guilt' and 'a need for punishment' (Freud, 1961 [1923], p. 49). Like Crystalman's 'sordid bestial grin', they cast 'a cold shadow of moral nastiness into every heart' (Lindsay, 1920, p. 18). The 'moral nastiness' of superego results in a brutal melancholia – a plight which Freud evocatively describes:

> The patient represents his ego to us as worthless, incapable of any achievement and morally despicable; he reproaches himself, vilifies himself and expects to be cast out and punished.
>
> (Freud, 1917, p. 246)

Evil and the 'Mystery Man'

The evil/vulgar grin is a trope which permeates horror cinema and is brilliantly deployed in David Lynch's ecstatic noir *Lost Highway* (1997). The central character, Fred Madison, soon to be accused of his wife's murder, meets 'the mystery man' at a party who also bears the satanic, painted grin of a clown. In the short scene when he first appears, his black, piercing eyes betray nothing but evil intent as he smiles manically at Madison. The sonic landscape which the two inhabit quickly transforms from 90s lounge trip-hop through a warped, liminal atonality into the foreboding buzzing drones of factory machinery, the call of an industrialised *maleficium*.

The party continues unabated, but the other guests are swiftly rendered nebulous ghosts as Madison's now manifest unconscious takes centre stage. Time has stopped for him, and there is now no escape from his reckoning. The mystery man tells him that they have met before at Madison's house, and much to the latter's befuddled terror, the man informs him that he is also there 'right now'. Despite Madison's increasingly desperate protests, the mystery man – all the while maintaining his manic grin – hands him a huge mobile phone and instructs him to call home. This dramatic tension serves as a precursor to a moment of twisted catharsis when the mystery man's double answers the phone. Despite Madison's protests – alluding to atavistic vampire lore of 'letting the right one in' – the double informs him that he never goes where he is not invited. The doubling is confirmed by the simultaneous cackling of the mystery man and his *doppelgänger* as the imaginary is now punctured by the real (Lacan, 2006). One may interpret the mystery man as an embodiment of the 'shadow side of the psyche', the evil which is disowned – the aspect in Madison which would goad him into killing his wife (Jung 1966, p. 49). Nonetheless, it is not clear at this point in the film whether Madison is guilty or these are murderous phantasies fuelled by jealousy. The shadow is thus analogous to a malignant superego that punishes Madison's ego with the same veracity *as if he had* murdered his wife. This essential distinction is made by Freud in *Civilisation and Its Discontents*:

> an evil deed is on a par with evil intention; hence the consciousness of guilt and the need for punishment.
>
> (Freud, 2002, p. 82)

At the level of unconscious phantasy, therefore, intent and deed are the same and deserve the same punishment. In the curse position, the individual is always 'at fault' (guilty), has 'let the wrong one in' (evil), and is tortured by this each day. From this position, despite the knowledge of trauma, the individual feels guilty for being weak or foolish enough to have let the evil spirit in at all. It is this creeping narrowness in perception between reality and phantasy, guilt and evil which are potential avenues that lead from neurosis to psychosis and suicidality, starkly illustrating the potentially fatal relationship between the conjunction of guilt and evil.

A Case Vignette: Reverse Clowns

Mr. F. is a middle-aged man in weekly psychotherapy. This session takes place after six months of treatment.

Mr. F. is the youngest of three children. His mother was a successful painter whom he described as 'bohemian'. Mr. F. felt that his mother had always placed her artistic endeavours before her family. Mr. F. felt that his father, who worked as an engineer, had resented and envied his mother at times and felt side-lined by her artistic career. Mr. F.'s mother would also belittle his father for having a boring and unadventurous job. Mr. F. described his father as emotionally cold, and this sometimes made Mr. F. feel on edge around him, picking up on a latent aggression in his body language.

Mr. F.'s mother read tarot cards for friends and family members and had done readings for him on a few occasions when he was an adult, but he had taken it 'with a pinch of salt', as the readings always seem to divine that he would become successful as an artist and 'follow in her footsteps'. This made Mr. F. feel under pressure even though his mother had always emphasised that she only wanted him to 'follow his dreams' – whatever they were. He had tried art at school but had always preferred computers in the end. Eventually, after a brief stint at art college, Mr. F. settled on a career in technology. Yet his mother's ambitions for him had left him with a sense of guilt that he had let her down.

Although Mr. F. had wanted to go to the local comprehensive secondary school with his friends, his parents had insisted that he go to the same private school as his mother had attended, which specialised in the arts. Mr. F. found the transition from primary school difficult, and already crippled by shame because of his worsening facial acne, he was repeatedly called 'pizza face' by other children in his class. He spoke in one session of his father's frustration and lack of empathy when he told him about the name calling, even on one occasion questioning whether Mr. F. had been washing his face properly. His father once humiliated Mr. F. by drunkenly making jokes at his expense about his skin at a family gathering. Mr. F. learned at school that the only way to stop the bullying was to make others laugh – at which he became adept – yet he also felt that this new persona had all but taken over his personality, and much of the time, the jokes were at his own expense anyway.

In one session, Mr. F. spoke candidly of an Oedipal phantasy: that he would have liked to have ousted his father by becoming the man that his mother had wanted his father to be, yet, instead of his following in his mother's footsteps, he thought that he was now doing an 'updated version' of his father's job.

Mr. F. was now married with two teenage children and struggling with feeling isolated from them and his wife. He said that he wanted therapy to help him to reconnect with them, 'get back to his creative side', and perhaps change careers.

In today's session, Mr. F. was my first client of the day, and he had been waiting outside in the cold wintry morning for 15 minutes before I could let him in. As I had no waiting room, I had told Mr. F. at the beginning of therapy that he should arrive as close to time as possible, as I would not be able to let him in before then. Nevertheless, I noticed that Mr. F.'s early arrival had made me feel anxious, and I wondered what this was about. I then began to consider whether I should not just let him in early, particularly as it was so cold outside. It seemed punitive to not let him earlier, as it was 'only' five minutes after all. Yet then I reminded myself of our agreement and decided to keep to that.

Given the potency of my countertransference, I deemed it important to ask Mr. F. how it had been to wait outside in the cold at the beginning of the session. He told me that he thought that it was always important to arrive on time, as it wouldn't be 'professional' to show up late. He paused for a moment and laughed to himself. He said that he felt like he sounded like he was still at work and rolled his eyes theatrically. I felt that he wanted me to join in with something but wasn't yet sure what. After some moments, Mr. F. added that he *always* felt like he was at work, and his eyes and slightly quavering voice communicated a sense of dejection and sadness. Mr. F. then began to look uncomfortable, as if not knowing what to say, and suddenly affected the persona of a manic comedian: 'I may as well just break out the laptop and do a PowerPoint presentation now, eh?' He comedically mimed the motion of a laptop opening and even made an accompanying 'clicking' sound, as if it were all part of a vaudeville routine. Although I sensed that this had been a defensive manoeuvre, I found it funny and could not help but laugh. Suddenly, the punitive anxiety I had felt when Mr. F. arrived early returned, and I wondered whether I 'should' have been laughing along with Mr. F., as it seemed that this impromptu performance had been a way of alleviating his anxiety. Was I colluding with a bad object? Although I had held the earlier boundary by not opening the door early, by laughing, I now felt that I had become an *accomplice* in Mr. F.'s self-denigrating routine. Mr. F. sat back in his chair and looked downcast and confused.

'I don't know what that was all about', Mr. F. said with a smile, but the sense of dejection had returned to his voice.
'What do you make of it?' I asked.
'I'm not sure really'. He continued to look lost. 'I'm doing it again aren't I?'
'What's that?' I asked, wishing to emphasise a gentleness in my curiosity.
'Making jokes when I feel anxious'.
I thought for a few moments and decided that a direct response would only concretise his experience. It struck me as important to work with the emerging symbolic content.
'Well, I was wondering whether you wanted to present something here today in some way?' I asked. I wanted to convey that I understood the need for this defence but that I wished to think with him about what this was defending against.
He laughed again, this time ruefully, and thought for a few moments. 'Yeah, I guess so, in a way it seems like a job interview or like I'm auditioning for a part . . . but it's actually probably my way of saying I think I'm boring, and I feel embarrassed about it. I try to make up for that by making people laugh'.
'How did you feel when I laughed?'
'Good for a moment [he looked down hesitantly], but then it's like you *have to* laugh, a bit like my kids do when I tell "dad jokes". . .'.

I knew how much Mr. F. loved his children, and for a moment I felt profoundly
moved by the look of pathos in his eyes and his gentle snort when he said
'dad jokes'. It made me think about what a great dad Mr. F. must be to his
kids. Yet there was an accompanying resignation in his voice, and again I
felt a pang of shame for laughing at his 'presentation'.

'I was wondering if you could say more about why I would *have to* laugh?'
I asked.

Mr. F. frowned. 'Maybe you don't want to be unkind? I dunno'.

Ahh, OK. 'So it's kinder to pretend?'

'Well yeah, I guess. I don't want to hurt other people's feelings. I just want
other people to be happy, I guess'.

'So you felt that I was laughing just to keep you happy?' I asked. There was a
prolonged pause.

'Basically yeah'.

'What do you think I was really thinking?'

'I dunno. Maybe that I'm a sad person? I wouldn't be here otherwise, would I?
People are laughing at me rather than with me'. The dejected look returned,
but then looked animated, even excited by his thoughts.

'It's weird. This reminds me of a dream I had as a teenager that I haven't
thought about for years'.

The Dream

*I'm at the circus with my wife and kids, and we're watching clowns do their routine
in the ring, walking on stilts and riding around on those little cars like they do. The
audience is laughing like crazy, and I'm laughing hysterically too, but then it all
starts to feel too much, and I begin to feel a bit panicky, and I want it to stop. I turn
to my wife next to me for reassurance, but she's now wearing a clown's outfit, and
everyone's got this evil clown grin. So I then turn to my kids, and they are too. That
was horrific. I then notice that everyone in the circus is now a clown. I start to feel
really panicked and looking down at my clothes I can see that I'm the only one in
the whole circus who isn't a clown – I've got my work suit on. The scene suddenly
switches, and I'm looking in a mirror and I'm snarling at myself – I look evil. I'm
then back in the circus, but I'm right there in the middle of the ring alone. Every
single seat in the circus is occupied by a clown roaring with laughter. I feel terrified
but also somehow guilty that I've left my family alone to be taken by the clowns.
The dread is overwhelming, and I wake up. The thing is, though, when I wake up,
I can see there's a dark mass in the corner of the room and I get that same sense
of dread that was there at the end of the dream. The mass morphs into a silhouette
of a body, and in the darkness, I can just about make out a face and its eldritch
smile – I say 'its' cos I have no idea what 'it' is. I'm frozen to the bed, and I pull
the sheets up around me until I get the courage to switch the light on. Of course,
when I do there's nothing there. I just remember thinking that I knew that I'd met
the Devil himself.*

I asked Mr. F. what he remembered about what was happening in his life when he'd had the dream. He said that he thought he was probably around 13 or 14 but didn't really remember much about that time. He thought for a while to himself before recalling being awoken one night around that time by loud 60s music as his parents were having a party. He recalled his mother 'raucously' laughing with her friends, and that there was something 'witchy' about her. She was wearing 'flowing 70s robes', and his father stared at her resentfully.

'So, what do you make of this dream now?' I asked. 'Do you think there was any connection between this memory of the party and the dream?'

'Not that I can think of', Mr. F. replied.

I decided to tell him my own observation, as the link seemed important. 'The way you described the clowns' laughter reminded of the way you described your mother laughing at the party somehow'.

'Ahh yes!' replied Mr. F. with enthusiasm. 'I can see that now! Something evil somehow'.

'You feel that your mum's expectations of you are evil?' I asked

'Well, evil might be a bit much [he laughed], but I don't think it's done me much good'.

'Do you think it's influenced your expectations of yourself?'

'One hundred percent', he replied, with increasing urgency and determination. 'Somehow I need to find a way to stop this thing of trying to be the clown', he continued. 'I'm tired of trying to impress other people. I am beginning to realise what's important. I don't actually care about being "creative". It's not necessary, is it? Yeah, my job isn't exciting, but I enjoy it well enough, and I love my family, so to be honest I don't really care whether my mum doesn't think it's right for me. I think my dad couldn't stand up to my mum, so he put all his shit onto me, and that's hard to forgive, but I won't be defined by that anymore. I don't want to be a victim'.

Mr. F. looked across at me, partially frowning in reflection, his eyes quietly yet determinedly resolute.

Discussion

This case illustration demonstrates the danger that one's ego-ideal – *daimonic* spirit/individuation – can become crushed by the ideal-ego/superego. From the beginning of the session, I could see Mr. F.'s anxieties around boundaries. He wanted to appear 'professional' by arriving early to assuage his anxieties around the threatening chaos of the superego that quickly became evident. I quickly came to embody an arbiter of the ideal-ego[5]/superego, judging him for job interview/audition, and had the power to decide whether he was funny or not. The wounded part of Mr. F. hoped that I would laugh along with him and accept him, yet was also ashamed that he knew that he was identifying with an ideal which was not really his own and was also frightened that I might shame him the way that his father had. I also felt this shame in the countertransference that I colluded with the bad object which crushed his potential, identified with his internalised mother's ideal-ego and his father's cruel superego.

Our exploration of the symbol of the 'presentation' proved to be beneficial, as it unlocked Mr. F.'s unconscious associations with his teenage dream and the party. Mr. F.'s anxiety around the threatening insecurity of boundaries resurfaced in the dream as he experienced the violent transition from spectator to become the humiliated subject of the spectacle, being mocked by multiple representations of the ideal-ego. At the beginning of the dream, the clowns safely embodied his shame and ridicule of the failed ideal-ego, but this collapsed as he saw a vision of his wounded, snarling self in the looking glass. His reflected double embodied all the shame, guilt and evil of his culpevility: of not following in his mother's footsteps, his father's humiliating jibes, and his betrayal of his own *daimonic* spirit. The combined evil and guilt of culpevility, however, proved unbearable to Mr. F.'s ego, and the evil was thus projected into the clown crowd, who persecuted him with the mirth identified with his father's mockery – the same mirth that Mr. F. had projected into me as a spectator when Mr. F. became the spectacle of his 'presentation'. Mr. F.'s dread of this evil was so unbearable that it could not be contained within the confines of the dream and then haunted him in his bedroom – like an incubus – and became the 'Devil himself'.

It is clinically important to note that Mr. F.'s unconscious had also autonomously made a link between the 'evil' of the clowns' 'roaring' laughter and his 'witchy', 'raucous' mother's by making these memories conscious. Mr. F.'s recollection of his father's resentment in the party memory was also significant, as he could then access his own resentful feelings towards the narcissistic eye identified with his mother. By making the connection between the manifest content of the dream and its associated party memory, Mr. F. had been presented with a temporal indication of the genesis of the pathological ideal and its link to his disconnection from his family and his *daimonic* spirit.

Concluding Comments

This chapter has illustrated the way in which one's narcissistic wounds and the ideals of one's parents can build up unachievable ideals, which can become persecutory and corrode one's legitimate ambitions. The mythologies of Prometheus and Narcissus demonstrate the way that one can become blind and confuse daimonic spirit with pathological narcissism. We have also seen the way in which the ideal-ego, when combined with relational trauma, becomes an impossible and persecutory ideal through which the individual deludes oneself that one's parents' love and acceptance can be regained.

Notes

1 Freud uses the term 'ideal-ego' interchangeably with 'ego-ideal' when he first introduces the concept in 1914's *On Narcissism*, which can be confusing. I have therefore found the 1963 paper by Sandler et al. to be extremely helpful in providing enlightening clarification.

2 In the earliest months, these are proto-object representations – see Beebe and Lachmann (1988) and Chapter 3.
3 These are the superego, id, and external reality. See Freud, 1973 [1932].
4 This indicates a desire to have what the other has, rather than its classical meaning of defence.
5 From here on, I use 'ideal-ego' to indicate the pathological ego-ideal, following Hanly's model (1984).

References

Beebe, B. and Lachmann, F. M. (1988). The contribution of mother-infant mutual influence to the origins of self- and object representations. *Psychoanalytic Psychology,* 5(4): 305–337.

Bloom, H. (1982). *Agon. Towards a Theory of Revisionism.* Oxford: Oxford University Press.

Fairbairn, R. (1943 [1952]). The Repression and the Return of Bad Objects (with Special Reference to the War Neuroses). In W. R. Fairbairn (ed), *Psychoanalytic Studies of the Personality.* London: Routledge and Kegan Paul.

Ferenczi, S. (1988). Confusion of tongues between adults and the child – The language of tenderness and of passion. *Contemporary Psychoanalysis,* 24: 196–206.

Freud, S. (1914). On Narcissism. In Freud, A., Strachey, A., Strachey, J, and Tyson A. (Eds.), *The Standard Edition of the Complete Psychological Works of Sigmund Freud, Volume XIV (1914–1916): On the History of the Psycho-Analytic Movement, Papers on Metapsychology and Other Works.* London: The Hogarth Press and the Institute of Psychoanalysis, pp. 67–102.

Freud, S. (1915). Instincts and their vicissitudes. *SE,* 14: 109–140.

Freud, S. (1917). Mourning and Melancholia. In Freud, A., Strachey, A., Strachey, J, and Tyson A. (Eds.), *The Standard Edition of the Complete Psychological Works of Sigmund Freud, Volume XIV (1914–1916): On the History of the Psycho-Analytic Movement, Papers on Metapsychology and Other Works,* London: The Hogarth Press and the Institute of Psychoanalysis, pp. 237–258.

Freud, S (1961 [1923]). The Dependent Relationships of the Ego. In J. Strachey (ed), *The Standard Edition of the Complete Psychological Works of Sigmund Freud, Volume XIX (1923–1925): The Ego and the Id and Other Works.* London: The Hogarth Press and the Institute of Psychoanalysis, pp. 1–308.

Freud, S. (1973 [1917]). Lecture 26, *Libido Theory and Narcissism in Volume 1, Introductory Lectures on Psychoanalysis: Pelican.* London: Reading and Fakenham.

Freud, S. (1973 [1932]). Lecture 26, *Psychical Dissection of the Personality in Volume 1, Introductory Lectures on Psychoanalysis: Pelican.* London: Reading and Fakenham.

Freud, S. (2002). *Civilization and its Discontents.* London: Penguin.

Hanly, C. (1984). Ego-ideal and Ideal ego. *The International Journal of Psychoanalysis,* 65(3): 253–261.

Jung, C. G. (1966). *Two Essays on Analytical Psychology* (2nd edn. rev. and augmented [by two appendices discovered among Jung's posthumous papers]). Princeton and London: Princeton University Press; Routledge and Kegan Paul.

Kanzer, M. (1964). Freud's uses of the terms "Autoerotism" and "Narcissism". *Journal of the American Psychoanalytic Association,* 12(3): 529–539.

Kohut, H. (1966). Forms and transformations of Narcissism. *Journal of the American Psychoanalytic Association,* 14: 243–272.

Lacan, J. and Fink, B. (2006). *Ecrits: The First Complete Edition in English*. New York: W.W. Norton & Co.

Lindsay, D. (1920). *A Voyage to Arcturus*. London: Penguin Classics.

Lynch, D. and Gifford, B. (1997). *Lost Highway*. October Films.

Muller, J. (1985). Lacan's mirror stage. *Psychoanalytic Inquiry: A Topical Journal for Mental Health Professionals*, 5(2): 233–252.

Perera, S. (1986). *The Scapegoat Complex: Toward a Mythology of Shadow and Guilt*. Toronto: Inner City Books.

Sandler, J., Holder, A. and Meers, D. (1963). The ego-ideal and the ideal self. *Psychoanal Study Child*, 18: 139–158.

Winnicott, D. W. (1960). The theory of the parent-infant relationship. *International Journal of Psychoanalysis*, 41: 585–595.

Winnicott, D. W. (2005). Mirror-Role of Mother and Family in Child Development. In Winnicott (ed.) *Playing and Reality*. London: Routledge.

Chapter 9

The Evil Eye & Limited Good

The Evil Eye owns two-thirds of the graveyard.

—Moroccan proverb

Introduction

This chapter researches the concept of 'the evil eye' in the context of the anthropological concept of 'the image of limited good'. These combined concepts form an epistemological base from which I examine the psychological, socioeconomic, and political power relations that contribute to the curse position, with particular regard to envy and hostility. Folkloric beliefs in the evil eye, witchcraft, and occult cursing practices have, since ancient times, become sources of revenge and agency by the oppressed as a means of addressing subjugation by the oppressor. These social disparities are illustrated through anthropological and historical research concerning the Ethiopian *buda*, the Tanzanian Azande, and Thomas Hardy's short story 'The Withered Arm'. Jessica Benjamin's concept of 'rational violence' offers a complementary feminist and psychoanalytic perspective to Emma Wilby's historical research into witchcraft, with particular regard to the Western Enlightenment's rejection of subjective, magical consciousness in favour of rationalist positivism. The chapter contains a case illustration concerning the envious evil eye and its related vicissitudes of transference and countertransference phenomena.

The Gaze

As Chapter 2 illustrated, there are overlaps between affective and telepathic phenomenology, and this may provide an explanation for the *uncanny* nature of the gaze. Building on this, the previous chapter has shown how the specular ego-ideal *haunts* the subject in the form of a spectral double. The ego-ideal's gaze is uncanny, as it may not be all that it first seems and is therefore 'anamorphic' (Lacan and Miller, 2008).

The gaze's spectral quality evokes the convergence of 'the weird and the eerie', as its presence persists in its absence (Fisher, 2016). As Lacan affirms, even

DOI: 10.4324/9781003168027-10

in blindness one knows that he remains the object of the gaze (Lacan and Miller, 2008). Many of us are familiar with the uncanny feeling that we are being stared at and then turn around to find that it is indeed the case (Sheldrake, 2005).

The eyes betray subtle cues of what we feel, much of which is beyond our conscious control. Research demonstrates that in both humans and animals, eyes 'are the most accurately decoded aspect of the face' (Bever, 2008, p. 25). Most therapists would now acknowledge the importance of nonverbal communication in countertransference, yet it is easy to forget that this is a two-way process/mirror; it is intersubjective. The gaze becomes particularly significant when one considers that when ocular activity is perceived in the therapist, this leads to an 'autonomic adjustment' and emotional response in the client, and *vice versa without conscious awareness* (ibid.; italics my own). Importantly, this spontaneous and unconscious autonomic adjustment applies to all human interaction (ibid.).

The Evil Eye

We might think about the evil eye as an arcane antecedent of the gaze. Evidence of belief in the evil eye is found in Ancient Babylonian, Egyptian, Greek, and Indian civilisations and is therefore believed to be widespread (Lykiardopoulos, 1981). The evil eye is a form 'of malign sight' that is often part of the beholder's 'possessing constitution', which means that they are unconscious of its effects and cannot therefore be held responsible for the injury caused to the recipient (Hutton, 2017, p. 10). According to Hutton, where belief in witchcraft is prevalent, there is a corresponding absence of belief in the evil eye, and the concepts are generally used mutually exclusively as explanations for uncanny misfortune (Hutton, 2017, p. 11). Like witchcraft, the gaze of the evil eye is to be feared, as it indicates hostility, envy, or even death.

Anthropologists conceptualise the evil eye as a result of 'the image of limited good', a concept formed out of the fieldwork of George M. Foster in Latin American, European, and African 'peasant' communities in the 1960s who perceived

> their social, economic, and natural universes – their total environment as one in which all of the desired things in life such as land, wealth, health, friendship and love, manliness and honor, respect and status, power and influence, security and safety, exist in finite quantity and are always in short supply.
>
> (Foster, 1965, p. 296)

Thus, from the worldview of 'the image of limited good', due to the finite nature of resources, personal gain is potentially detrimental to one's neighbour. This applies to families too: the jealousy evoked in siblings and fathers at the arrival of a new baby is attributed to the perceived limited nature of a mother's love, none of which is intentional but a matter of *fate* (ibid.; Hutton, 2017). Complementing other members of the community is therefore perceived as a threat, as it is an indicator of the *covetous envy* of the evil eye (Foster, 1965).

For Melanie Klein, envy is a developmentally oral and projective phenomenon. The 'evil eye' exists in the infant's unconscious or the mother's breast. Through envy of the breast, the infant sets out

> to put badness, primarily bad excrements and bad parts of the self, into the mother, and first of all into her breast, in order to spoil and destroy her. In the deepest sense this means destroying her creativeness.
>
> (Klein, 1997, p. 181)

Due to the re-creation of family dynamics that recur in the transference and the primitive feelings of powerlessness that this can evoke, envious attacks on therapists are therefore to be expected.

The *Buda* of Ethiopia

Aside from the immediacy of the influence of family dynamics on the transference, it is also important to consider the way in which hierarchical social class structures play a significant role in determining societal and individual perceptions of the evil eye. Finneran (2003) points out that although anthropologists have focused on the envy of the 'have-nots' in communities, the attribution of the *malocchio* to those with less economic wherewithal also symbolically maintains the superior status quo for the 'haves' as part of engrained, regulating social systems which Bordieu conceptualises as 'habitus' (1977). As will become clear later in the chapter, the concept of the 'image of limited good' is a useful means of thinking about a sense of existential finitude in communities and in unconscious phantasy.

The evil eye is an important injunctive image of limited good in societies where those with fewer material resources at their disposal both envy and present a threat to those who possess them. Like the gaze, it is therefore present even in absence. As resources in limited-good societies are considered part of a zero-sum equation, the evil eye of envy is thus potently cathected. With this in mind, I now give an example of how the evil eye serves as a means of demarcating two classes of people in the Ethiopian highlands as part of a limited-good kinship system.

Amharan society contains Monophysite Christian, pagan, and animistic entities (Reminick, 1974; Baynes-Rock, 2015). The landowning Amhara people perceive themselves to be *rega* (nobility) who possess a superior status to the landless *buda*, who are not indigenous to the region and typically earn a living as artisans such as tanners, blacksmiths, and weavers (Reminick, 1974, p. 289). The *buda* are believed by the Amhara to possess the evil eye and –which is perhaps more difficult to comprehend from a typically Global Northern perspective – also to be supernatural entities with independent consciousness. They are therefore both humans and familiar spirits. In the case of the Amhara, as they believe the *buda* to be envious of their regal social stature, there is always a danger that they will become the victims of a magically driven envious attack (Baynes-Rock, 2015, p. 266).

According to Amharan beliefs, the *buda* are a people who have been cursed by God as punishment for the sins of Eve,[1] and each new generation therefore inherits this tragic malediction. This curse renders the *buda* scapegoated 'agents of the Devil' who possess an unconscious satanic power called *qalb*, which is the font of the hostile power of the evil eye (Reminick, 1974, pp. 283–286). The *buda* are also believed to have further magical abilities such as astral travel, shapeshifting into hyenas, and 'eating'[2] their human prey, resulting in disease or death (Reminick, 1974, p. 281). This 'eating' therefore also symbolises an important levelling of the social class playing field (Galt, 1982, p. 667).

Along with the shapeshifting powers of the *buda*, they also can ride and harness hyenas as familiars to attack their human prey (Baynes-Rock, 2015, p. 274). Hyenas can also be 'employed' to exhume Amhara corpses from the graveyard, which the *buda* will then reanimate for employment as revenant familiars or slaves, thereby once again reversing the power dialectic with the Amhara[3] (Reminick, 1974, p. 283). There are clearly parallels here with the spirit familiars of Western witchcraft. Indeed, the capacity of the *buda* to night-ride on the spirit realm is reminiscent of popular European witchcraft lore where witches ride various animals, shapeshift into them, use them as familiars, or animate objects for astral travel. Inanimate objects such as the witch's broomstick are brought to demonic life by spiritualising them with the 'balm of the Devil', which thus bears some similarity to the *qalb* (Hutton, 2017). The capacity for 'astral' or 'soul' travel is also well documented in the witchcraft of the Azande tribe of North Central Africa; the 'soul' takes the form of a bright light which also is an omen of hostile intent to the recipient: the light represents the *mbisimo mangu*, or the 'soul of witchcraft' (Evans-Pritchard, 1976, p. 10).

> The soul of witchcraft may leave its corporeal home at any time during the day or night, but Azande generally think of a witch sending his soul on errands by night when his victim is asleep. It sails through the air emitting a bright light. During the daytime this light can only be seen by witches, and by witch-doctors when they are primed with medicines, but anyone may have the rare misfortune to observe it at night.
>
> (Evans-Pritchard, 1976, p. 11)

The Azande also say that 'witchcraft is like fire, it lights a light'. The 'light' therefore represents the spiritualised psychic realm that can only be apprehended during the day by witch doctors through the ingestion of hallucinogenic plants. For the rest of the community, witnessing the light happens only at night within the confines of nightmare. This Azande light, *buda qalb*, or witches' Devil's balm all represent hostile intent. Yet they also help the witch/*buda* transcend the confines of the phenomenal self by facilitating soul travel or by 'becoming' an animal double – not the subservient double of Lacan's specular ideal-ego but one which can be *employed* as a collaborative ally. The 17th century testimony of Isobel Gowdie documents her capacity to shapeshift into hares, jackdaws, and crows. Such therianthropic powers meant Gowdie could access the houses of the wealthy and enjoy their high-quality food and beverages (Callow, 2018, p. 135).

These examples illustrate how beliefs associated with magical abilities such as the evil eye, soul travel, and shapeshifting are intertwined with complex social systems concerned with scarcity of resources, the management of social and economic disparity, and the concomitant envy and aggression.

'The Withered Arm'

Cultural factors which coalesce around the evil eye, such as envy and uncanny misfortune, are important aspects of Thomas Hardy's late 19th century short story 'The Withered Arm'. The story presents a stark depiction of the tragically repressive taboos of a 'limited-good' village in 19th century rural west-country England, a setting infused with folklore and grim, fatalistic superstition. Rhoda Brook, the middle-aged protagonist of the story, is a milkmaid who lives in the village with her son. The son's father is Farmer Lodge, though the reader is left to assume that Lodge has abandoned the pair and that the birth was out of wedlock. Lodge has recently married the much younger Gertrude, and Rhoda is consumed with jealousy. She begins to develop phantasies about Gertrude which reach a point of nocturnal catharsis when the latter visits her as an *incubus* as she sleeps:

> . . . the young wife, in the pale silk dress and white bonnet, but with features shockingly distorted, and wrinkled by age, was sitting upon her chest as she lay. The pressure of Mrs Lodge's person grew heavier; the blue eyes peered cruelly into her face, and then the figure thrust forward its left hand mockingly, so as to make the wedding-ring it wore glitter in Rhoda's eyes.
>
> (Hardy, 1976, p. 71)

Here, Rhoda's own maligned aspects (distorted wrinkled features, age) painfully interact with the idealised objects of her envied rival double (pale silk dress, wedding ring). In her fury and terror, Rhoda then seizes 'the confronting spectre by its obtrusive left arm', which is what is to result in the withered arm that gives the story its title (ibid.). Despite all of the apparent mutually expressed aggression in the nightmare rendezvous, Rhoda is subsequently consumed with guilt following a 'real-life' encounter with Gertrude two weeks later. Rhoda realises that the nocturnal attack coincided precisely with the onset of Gertrude's now withered arm, which the latter cannot account for as she conveys no memory of the nightmare meeting. Although the incubus nightmare is over, Rhoda is now confronted by the new horror of the daylight realities of her own aggression: the sheer force of her projected hostility into the visiting *imago* could not be contained by the confines of the nightmare and resulted in Gertrude's morbid affliction. For Rhoda, this represents a confirmation that it is she, not Gertrude, who possesses the 'malignant' power of the *incubus*: one that 'had been slily called a witch since her fall'[4] (Hardy, 1976, p. 75).

Rhoda's cognizance of the withered arm means that she can no longer use Gertrude as a container for her aggression, and she is now beset by persecutory thoughts. In an attempt to help her afflicted rival, Rhoda then recommends that Gertrude consult a 'white wizard' known as 'Conjuror Trendle', who informs her that the wound is the result of a supernatural attack, and, much to her shock, his scrying glass reveals Rhoda to be the culprit. Gertrude's husband Lodge now abandons her when she needs him most. He rejects her out of narcissistic necessity: she is no longer sexually desirable to him, and he is troubled that she is consulting cunning folk and trusting in herbal remedies.

Gertrude visits Trendle again 'in a last desperate effort at deliverance from this seeming curse', and he tells her that the only way to heal the wound is by 'turning the blood' by pressing her arm against the neck of a hanged man 'before he's cold, just after he's cut down' (Hardy, 1976, p. 84). In a devastating finale, Gertrude comes to realise that the hanged man who was to unknowingly provide the antidote was Rhoda and Lodge's son. Gertrude then dies shortly after the hanging episode, and Rhoda's life ebbs away from her in abject poverty. Lodge continues to prosper financially, and although he subsequently shows remorse for his actions, it is only when it is too late.

While reflecting on the events that lead to the story's tragic end, I cannot help wondering how things would have been different had Lodge not abandoned everyone he was supposed to have taken care of and whether these tragic events would have occurred at all. It may on the surface seem surprising, therefore, that Rhoda does not reserve more of this hostility for Lodge, yet perhaps not when one considers the societal strictures to which she was bound. Rhoda, as a daughter of Eve, like the cursed *buda*, is a sinner of the fall; she is doomed to carry the sins of those with the power and agency from which she is excluded. It is important to note that when Rhoda meets Gertrude in her nightmare, she is described as an *incubus* rather than a *succubus*, the former of which is typically attributed to a male demonic entity. Hardy's incongruous use of the term then informs the reader – perhaps purely due to *lapsus* on the author's part – that, indeed, it is Lodge who is the true object of Rhoda's hostility, the *actual incubus* of the tale, yet, as he can only be perceived in noble and virtuous terms, his demonic aspect is projected into Gertrude. Hardy's *lapsus* therefore – perhaps unintentionally – becomes a meta-participation in denying Rhoda and Gertrude the aggressive aspects that belong to the *succubus* by replacing them with a demiurgic, male substitute. Rhoda is ergo rendered a Promethean demon stripped of her power; like the witches of the early modern period, she holds the toxins of society, yet she is denied the spoils of aggression, which are only reserved for powerful, narcissistic men such as Lodge. The evil eye in this tale, then, is neither Rhoda's nor Gertrude's but the cruel ocular superego of the society which subjugates them. In 'The Withered Arm', then, we have two women who are denied 'mutual recognition' – even in dreams – without the interference and intrusion of a male object (Benjamin, 1980). Rhoda's projection of her own withered aspects into Gertrude are therefore her only recourse to recognition, as she unconsciously knows that it is only with Rhoda that she may find the recognition that she desires. Lodge, in his abandonment of both women, emphasises his independence and difference, where both women in the story, despite their struggle for differentiation, are condemned to be the same.

> One posture, traditionally male, overemphasizes self boundaries and the other posture, traditionally female, over emphasizes the relinquishing of self. The splitting of these postures is the most important boundary of all.
>
> (Benjamin, 1980, p. 146)

Aside from the gender aspect that Benjamin importantly highlights here, it is also important for therapists to address such boundary issues and how they impact on therapeutic dyads and to explore both with their clients and in supervision how boundary constellations have evolved and play out in the transference. Clients, for example, presenting with preoccupied/borderline forms of relating will be more prone to relinquishing the self, where more schizoid, avoidant clients will tend to emphasise the boundary.

Rationalism as a Defence against Aggression in the Other

Jessica Benjamin's work continues to provide a contemporary psychoanalytic perspective today on power relations as when she wrote *The Bonds of Love* in 1980. As earlier chapters have illustrated, the subjugation of children's subjectivity is a major causative factor in the curse position. Clients who require connection, fluidity, and nurture are confronted by a culture which repetitively undermines selfhood through a divisive capitalist realism where profit and 'efficiency' precede and override nurture and connection, despite its frequent and empty claims to the contrary (Fisher, 2009). Benjamin's work thus emphasises the schism between 'rational' orthodoxies and the syncretic, non-Western epistemologies which are regarded by more fundamentalist representatives of the former as 'primitive' or 'irrational'. The fundamentalist aspect of rationalism is what Benjamin calls 'instrumentalism', which defers to 'objectivity', and is – I believe due to its inherent and wilful blindness – unable to hold the necessary tension between dependency and differentiation that is required in order to form a society which accepts heterodox ontologies. This rigid worldview maintains the cultural bounds of the image of 'limited good', where beliefs which diverge from phenomenal orthodoxy are quickly dismissed, driven by a primitive, narcissistic fear of annihilation in the subject.

> The most familiar conflict that arises from differentiation is between the need to establish autonomous identity and the need to be recognized by another. . . . This world view emphasizes difference over sameness, boundaries over fluidity. It conceives of polarity and opposition, rather than mutuality and interdependence,

as the vehicles of growth. That is, it does not tolerate the simultaneous experience of contradictory impulses: ambivalence.

(Benjamin, 1980, p. 148)

As Benjamin's work demonstrates, it is this paranoid-schizoid splitting process which ensures that that the powerful – through the 'instruments' of differentiation and rationality – maintain a position of control. For the traumatised subject who is already alienated from her own subjectivity, the continued brutal demarcation of rationalism results in an exponential depletion of agency which leads to despair: the traumatised subject collapses in a state of helplessness and shame (Ataria, 2015, p. 146). The contemporary 'solutions' offered in response to the collateral distress range from poorly funded industrialised public health services and/or soul-numbing pharmaceutical drugs to short-term manualised therapies designed to get people 'back to work'. The most horrifying aspect of this subjugating dialectic is that for those who are unable to 'benefit' from it, the only real means of differentiation becomes desperate flights from what Rhoda so evocatively called her 'seeming curse' into addiction, self-harm, and suicide. The *wyrd*/weird outsider archetype that is the DNA of the curse position is therefore a defensive means of reclaiming the differentiation that has been lost through the traumatic undermining of subjectivity. The subject experiences a psycho-somatic deficit that a core, vulnerable self has been tarnished or stolen from them, as in cases of violent or sexual abuse. Such trauma can lead to extreme states of psychic distress where it is the body that becomes a 'theatre of the self' that plays a central part in extreme enactments of differentiation such as with anorexia nervosa. In such cases, the body itself becomes a *memento mori* which, in its attempt to disappear and the construction of a 'no entry' defence, paradoxically attracts the gaze of the other which the subject experiences as a persecutory invader of her boundaries (Williams, 1997, p. 121).

We have seen in Chapter 3 the interplay of trauma and unconscious phantasy which contribute to the curse position. For the traumatised individual, the retreat into unconscious phantasy as a defence against the harmful aspects of relationship presents a limited-good–style conundrum: *to save oneself from harm from the other or keep the other safe from harmful parts of the self.* The absence of the possibility of forming meaningful and sustained relationships with professionals in the medical and care sectors can only compound the schizoid aspect of the individual, as society itself offers a schizoid form of care. Given this scenario, it is not difficult to see the appeal of the occult as a curative alternative, as it offers a sense of empowerment to the powerless. Esoteric and magical practices and levels of consciousness have become a means of expressing the aggressive and hostile aspects of the self which have hitherto been denied a voice, whether it be by institutions, societal values, or interfamilial relationships. As I have described in Chapters 3 and 4, the trauma experiences which haunt the cursed subject stem from the child's identification with her caregivers, and becoming 'clairvoyant' to the latter's needs forms a phantasy that this will not only help her avoid further abandonment, boundary violation, or basic neglect but also erase those of the past. As with the myth of Cassandra, the cursed subject has acquired mediumistic powers at an early age, knows too much too soon, and fatally ignores her prophecy. In this sense, the occult is an obvious natural home as an adult, and its associated esoteric spiritual practices importantly also offer other ways of being in the world besides the enduringly dominant culture of positivist, capitalist materialism. Esoteric and 'new-age' practices may address the deficit through contact with nature; divinatory practices such as cartomancy and astrology; and – perhaps most importantly of all with regard to trauma – with the body, through practices such as yoga and qi gong, which have been demonstrated to alleviate PTSD (Van der Kolk, 2015). From this perspective, esoteric practices offer novel ways of healing trauma and become a means of its sublimation. Yet, if the 'clairvoyant' subject does not find a way of processing and containing trauma, then she risks continuing to live at the behest of her unconscious phantasies. There is also a risk that she will re-enact her trauma by putting others' needs before her own or by responding to pressing omnipotent thoughts that her clairvoyant powers can rescue others from their own narcissistic wounds.

Those who practice the occult may have had to contend with the judgements of orthodox religion and the sometimes sneering contempt of forms of hyper-rationalism which invoke 'science' to discredit other ontologies. It is not a surprise, then, that those who have felt cursed in this way would like to get their revenge through uncanny means such as those employed by the *buda*, Azande, and Isobel Gowdie. One of the key themes of this chapter concerns the way in which we relate to aggression in ourselves and in the other and how attributing and/or denying hostility to the other becomes a means of undermining subjectivity by asserting difference in the way that Benjamin highlights. To illustrate this point, it is now widely accepted among historians that the witches' testimonies at the time of their trials in early modern Europe were the result of forced confessions by the manipulative agenda of demonologist churchmen (Callow, 2018; Hutton, 2017). However, as Emma Wilby argues, notwithstanding the demonologists' clear coercive agenda and use of forced confessions, this does not rule out the possibility that 'black magic'[5] such as cursing practises took place and questions why it has since become a taboo to suggest this (Wilby, 2013). Wilby's research therefore provides a complementary historical perspective to Benjamin's in that she also pinpoints a continuing cultural inclination within the post-Enlightenment West to idealise ways of being in the world which fall outside of the narrative which it has for itself prescribed.

> Post enlightenment mentalities, unschooled in the subjective reality of magical thinking, may find it easier to rationalize how an individual might slaughter in the heat of battle, or execute a child in response to the letter of the law, than rationalize how they could create a clay image and carefully roast it before a fire in order to cause the death of an enemy. In conclusion, it could be argued that despite all the scholarly attention which early modern witchcraft has received over the last fifty years, in some respects maleficent magic remains taboo.
>
> (Wilby, 2013, p. 150)

By following Wilby's argument, one can see that the rationalist Western paradigm then unconsciously may collude with the demonologists it criticises, though draws a boundary through denial rather than projection. The unconscious taboo denies the witch her *succubae*, demonic aspects, and renders her a 'manageable' de-potentiated object through the unsolicited 'cleansing' of her dark, aggressive aspects through the filter of rationalism. The unconscious installation of the aggression taboo into cultural subjects that fall outside of the Western rational paradigm also means that pernicious levels of aggression may continue to be enacted through the well-established 'civilised' means of advanced capitalism of projection and denial of subjectivity. Those who do not possess the required leverage of *habitus* are thus denied their basic right to express hostility in order to claim the subjectivity that has been denied them. In cases where aggression is accepted in 'the other', it is – as Wilby says – only done as a justified response to an attack, yet it is only those who are in positions of power that can make that judgement call and who wield the privilege to truly indulge in aggression *for its own sake*. It is also only the powerful who have the means to commit acts of indulgent aggression with impunity and who use denial as their main weapon of choice. The fully industrialised limited-good society, then, is one where certain affective experiences – such as the satisfying catharsis of aggression – are only reserved for those who are privileged enough to experience them. It is therefore the evil eye of capitalism that is the image of limited good, for it is the infinite desire it creates in its subjects that causes them to remain in the thrall of its inherent lack, for capitalism itself is empty (Lacan, 2006).

This cultural cleaving of the dark and light aspects of the subject also holds profound significance for the curse position, where an already split, traumatised individual feels morally 'bad' and wishes to extricate this part of herself yet is full of rage at the sense of injustice towards those whom she implicitly blames for putting her 'badness' there. Here again, the occult offers a means of sublimation and empowerment to her, yet if her traumatic wounds are not sufficiently tended to, she may easily be tempted to embrace its idealised 'love and light' aspects, mistaking empowerment for omnipotence, thereby re-enacting her childhood trauma by denying and disowning her own sadistic desires, identifying with one part object and denying its opposite.

Case Illustration: The Evil Eye of the One That Needs to Know

Ms. D. is a woman in her late 20s, presenting with 'crippling' anxiety, panic attacks, and insomnia. Ms. D. was the middle sister of three and had been aware of the scarcity of financial and emotional resources in her home since she was a child, particularly as childcare and illness had placed limitations on her mother's ability to work. Ms. D.'s mother also suffered from depressive episodes, and, as her own parents had been emotionally remote, she had found it difficult to show affection to her children.

Ms. D.'s father worked long hours and was often not at home, though she felt that he was physically and emotionally affectionate when he was and understood how she felt much better than her mother did. However, when her father was at home, it was rare that Ms. D. had any time alone with him, as her mother and sisters also needed his attention. Ms. D. said that she felt as if her mother had always been particularly demanding of her father's attention and rarely left the house, which she found 'suffocating'. As a child, she frequently had a nightmare of an 'evil crow' tapping at her bedroom window.

Ms. D. felt that when she was growing up there was scant emotional and financial security available to her and that she had to compete with her sisters for what was available to get her emotional needs met. When she was a teenager, as her elder sister had moved out and her younger sister was five years younger than her, she had spent a lot of her time caring for her mother. Her mother said that her illness was 'typical' of her bad luck, and she felt resentful and envious of women her age who had gone onto have successful careers. Ms. D.'s mother also resented her dependence on her daughters for her care and Ms. D.'s father's preoccupation with his career. She would often complain to Ms. D. that he was 'too nice' and that despite working so hard, he had never made the most of the opportunities he'd been offered. Ms. D.'s mother would also often talk about how guilty she felt about placing so much responsibility on Ms. D. at a young age, which made her feel that 'everything always ended up being about my mum'. Ms. D. had consequently found it difficult to sustain intimate relationships, as she perceived emotional attachment as the first step towards a burdensome dependence on her, though if she felt that partners were losing interest, she would quickly become obsessive and clingy.

Ms. D.'s mother was often preoccupied with a persecutory future and anxieties around the progression of her illness, and she had found holistic approaches such as homeopathic medicine and Reiki helpful to alleviate her chronic pain. Her mother also consulted a tarot reader from time to time, and Ms. D. had inherited her mother's interest in cartomancy, usually finding something in the spreads that meant something significant to her. Ms. D. had now decided to try psychotherapy, as she was facing a crisis that was focused on her work and felt helpless. Ms. D. worked in the technology sector, and although she was not currently enjoying her work, she said that she couldn't bear to think about being unemployed, mainly due to the financial risk this would have entailed, which also reminded her of the financial insecurity she experienced growing up. Like her mother, Ms. D. was often troubled by punitive thoughts that she had been given a disproportionate amount of bad luck and that others were 'always' more successful than her and led more interesting lives.

After just four weeks of therapy, Ms. D. asked whether I thought it might be better to come every two weeks instead of the weekly basis on which we had originally agreed. I said that I understood that having a dependable weekly session may feel bring up familiar and uncomfortable feelings of what we had previously discussed with regard to her feeling like a burden on others. Ms. D. thought about what I had said for few moments and replied that she hadn't seen it in that way but agreed that this 'could be the case'. She then laughed and shrugged her shoulders, adding, 'I do think that coming weekly seems like an arbitrary decision that therapists make, but whatever . . . let's stick with what we have then for the time being'.

The Following Illustration Is Taken from a Session Six Months Later.

Ms. D. told me that she had found sleeping difficult recently, as she had been worrying about work. She said that many of her colleagues were more 'ruthless' when it came to 'doing what needed to be done' to get promoted and acquire bigger salaries, and in this way, she was 'too nice', just like her father. Until recently, Ms. D. had enjoyed a positive relationship with her (male) boss, who valued her work greatly. Since a new (female) colleague had joined the company, Ms. D. began to feel threatened because it seemed to her that the colleague had now become the boss's 'favourite' and was consequently being offered 'exciting new projects' that Ms. D. would have previously been first in line for.

Ms. D. told me that due to the pressures of her current work situation, she had decided to consult her tarot reader again. The reader had informed her that the spread suggested that there was perhaps someone in her life who did not 'have her best interests at heart'. Ms. D. had concluded that the reading had therefore pointed to her colleague, not only due to the work situation but also because since her colleague had started at the company, things had begun to deteriorate for Ms. D. in other areas of her life. In the last two months alone, her boiler had broken down, her dog had become unwell, and she had also lost her expensive new phone on a night out. She said that she knew it 'sounded paranoid' but that there was something really 'nasty' about her colleague and that she 'couldn't help thinking' that she had placed a curse on Ms. D. She then laughed and said that she knew it wasn't '*really* true' (she made the 'scare quotes' gesture) but couldn't help making the connection between her colleague starting at the company and her recent run of bad luck.

Although I already knew that Ms. D. consulted a tarot reader from time to time and that doing so was important to her, I felt taken aback by this revelation. I then felt quickly defensive and affronted, as if telling me about this had been an attack on my competency as a therapist. I also felt quite envious of the tarot reader, with whom it seemed I was now being put into competition or might even be completely replaced by. Due to the powerful countertransference response, I was conscious of quickly participating in an enactment and therefore wanted to remain as curious as possible without appearing defensive. I then said that I was curious to know what it was about this particular situation that had made her feel it necessary to see her tarot reader. Ms. D. replied that this was different from the 'ordinary kind of situation that we usually cover', as she felt that there was 'something like witchcraft involved' and this was an area where the tarot reader 'really knew his stuff'. This comment felt like she was putting me down as a therapist, and I was now unwittingly placed in a competition with the tarot reader. Maybe I didn't 'know my stuff' as well as he did? I felt backed into a corner and as if whatever I said would sound pettily territorial and would have betrayed underlying countertransference feelings of inadequacy and envy. After some moments of sitting with them, I came to understand that Ms. D. had made an important communication by projective identification. Ms. D. was clearly feeling quite scared about what was happening to her at work, and this had triggered some intolerable primitive phantasies driven by envy and dependency which scared and overwhelmed her. I therefore said that I understood why she felt the need to see her tarot reader, and although a part of her felt it wasn't '*really*' true that her colleague was a witch, she couldn't help thinking that she was, and having both those parts in the same room felt overwhelming to her. Although she agreed that this made sense, and it appeared that this interpretation served well enough to hold her competing anxieties for now, it felt as if I had, in doing so, avoided confronting the way in which she had identified with the denigrating, 'witch' part object demonstrated by her attack on me and the therapy. This was a 'ruthless' bad object that was 'cursing' me in the transference and, at the same time, keeping Ms. D. in the emotionally 'crippling' victim/curse position of her mother. However, I decided it was most sensible not to confront this object at this stage, as this would have meant crossing a defensive boundary that Ms. D. really needed to maintain.

A couple of weeks later, Ms. D. told me – in a rather tentative and subdued fashion – that she had thought of a new creative technological solution at work which could 'revolutionise' the way of working there. I was struck by how at odds her nonverbal expressions were with the content of what she was telling me; her shoulders were hunched up, and she looked uncertain and vulnerable. There was an inertness to her posture which was set in radical contrast to the almost hyperbolic nature of the word 'revolutionise', which made me think about a *gauche* advertising slogan. I responded by saying – and resisting a troubling temptation to adopt an equally *gauche* 'enthusiastic' mirroring intonation – that this sounded like an important discovery for her, given the uncertainty she had been feeling about her place at work and her colleague. There were a few moments of pause, and Ms. D. now slowly unfolded her arms while clasping her outstretched hands in front of her, seeming to suppress a feigned nonchalant yawn. She then said quietly, though still looking downwards, 'Yes, maybe . . . but I don't want to tell you what it is'. As Ms. D. generally had quite a dry sense of humour, I initially presumed this to be a demonstration of this now. After a few more moments had elapsed, however, I began to suspect that I had been mistaken, as her facial expression had now become steadfastly serious, even grave somehow. I was somewhat taken aback by this, as Ms. D. also didn't tell me *why* she didn't want me to know, so it seemed that this too would have to remain a mystery for the time being at least – part of a cryptic guessing game where only Ms. D. knew the rules. Suddenly, I experienced the unsettling feeling that I had involuntarily been placed in the role of the one who *needs to know*, as if I were, like her envious colleague, *coveting* this information. As with the tarot scenario, I now felt as if I had been excluded from something exclusive which had taken on a mysterious and seductive quality: the *l'objet petit a* (Lacan, 2006).

I inwardly questioned why I felt like I *needed to know* – after all, this wasn't *really* the case, as technology wasn't something that particularly interested me. Yet I was again being prohibited from something which, by virtue of its occlusive nature, had become desirable in the countertransference. This created a confusing double bind, because if I continued to ask Ms. D. more about her project idea, this once again may have felt like I was disrespecting a boundary which she had firmly drawn. Yet were I to sidestep this issue, I would reject Ms. D.'s unconscious wish that the mystery continued. I felt stuck and decided to say nothing.

I then became aware of the dusk of the late winter afternoon rapidly turning into the dark of the evening and noticed that I was also starting to feel rather cold. I inwardly reprimanded myself for not turning the radiator on earlier on when I got to the consulting room before Ms. D. arrived. I then started to feel – and am struck by how neurotically – concerned that Ms. D. might also have noticed the drop in temperature and wondered whether I should check whether she would also like me to turn the radiator on. I then surmised that this would be another way of rescuing myself from the wintry affects of the double bind and decided against it, though the fact that I was willing to 'sacrifice' myself by remaining cold for the rest of the session didn't occur to me until later that evening. It now seemed that only one of us could escape being left out in the cold. In the midst of this frosty reverie, I then remembered what the tarot reader had said a couple of weeks previously. I then added that I appreciated that Ms. D. may, at some level, have felt that I, like her colleague, might be another person who did not have her best interests at heart. Ms. D. then said immediately and quickly, 'Yes, that's exactly why I don't want to tell you . . . you might steal my idea'.

Initially, I again had the initial sense that Ms. D. was 'joking', perhaps as a means of communicating her desire to exclude and annihilate the envious object in the transference but which gave her the option to subsequently re-frame it as a light-hearted quip. Yet it soon became abundantly clear that, again, she was not joking. She now rested her chin in her hands, as if she were holding herself together. It was clear that my speculative interpretation had awakened the frightened infant in her, who feared the 'evil eye' of the crow tapping on the window and her impinging mother, both of whom had come to life in the transference. I then said to her that I thought it had been so important that she told me this, and perhaps this situation at work was creating conflicting feelings of seeking approval from others but also feeling that they cannot be trusted and will always rob her in the end. I wondered also, though, whether on some level by not telling me she wanted to protect me from the feelings she would have towards me once she had told me. There could never be a situation where we both won: someone had to lose.

The room still felt cold, and I had now become aware of a real sense of loss in the space between us. Ms. D. leaned towards me in her chair and said that the reason she didn't want to tell me about her project was because – besides her fear that I would steal her idea – she '*knew*' that I would want to know what it was and that to not know this would make me suffer – that I would get a 'dose' of what it felt like to be excluded in the way that she had been at work. She said that she now felt bad saying that, because she thought that I 'seemed like a nice person' so maybe yes, it was true she was worried about hurting my feelings and wanting to protect me from that. I asked her what this feeling reminded her of. After considering this for a few moments, she said it reminded her of the way she felt at home when her mother 'interfered with everything she did' and although she 'hated her for that', she always felt guilty for it. I said that I imagined it must have been difficult to express feelings of anger or disappointment towards her father too for her fear that she might drive him away completely – she needed to protect him from that too. I could now see that she had tears in her eyes. After a few moments, she said, with a sense of defiance that she was 'tired of giving away things so easily, without thinking properly'. I asked her if she was glad she hadn't therefore told me what her project was. She then smiled broadly and replied with an emphatic 'Yeah, absolutely!'

Ms. D. then took a big sigh, which felt like a huge unburdening of anguish. I asked her whether today's session had given her any further perspective on what the tarot reader had said to her a couple of weeks ago, referring to her colleague and the curse. She paused again and moved her mouth until it settled somewhere between a grimace and a smile. Ms. D. said, 'I know that she isn't a bad person, and wants to get on, just like me, but that doesn't mean I have to like her'. She smiled. 'But that also doesn't make her an evil witch either, I guess'. I then said that it was understandably easier to think about her colleague's curse on her rather than think about her boss' responsibility for this situation. 'Maybe', she said. 'I can see now that he is far from innocent'.

Discussion

By turning Ms. D.'s colleague into a bad object, Ms. D. had been able to defend against her loathing of being dependent on the decisions of more powerful people in her life. The powerlessness and sense of humiliation that Ms. D. experienced in having to compete with her colleague for her boss's approval mirrored her need to compete with her siblings for her father's love. Due to the affective power that was invested in the mysterious object of desire in the transference and countertransference, the object became an 'image of limited good': in this paranoid-schizoid phantasy, only one member of the dyad could obtain and enjoy the gaze of the father/boss/therapist object (ideal-ego). This would be to the detriment of the 'cursed' other, who would be *left out in the cold* with their needs unmet.

In sustaining this defiant netherworld of holding on to the privileged knowledge of holding an idealised object, it meant that Ms. D. could experience the triumphant feelings that she felt had been hitherto denied to her. She would no longer need to tolerate the paralysing feelings of envy and dependency, as she had now projected these into me, phantasising of a blissful state where dependence no longer existed. Her colleague held the 'ruthless', 'witch' part object on her behalf, yet also unconsciously drove her desire to 'do what needed to be done' to get her sisters, mother, and colleague out of the way to have 'time alone' with her father/boss. Yet now, the 'time alone' with me became overwhelming to Ms. D. in the transference, and she therefore could only project her raw feelings into me, so that I had a 'dose' of what she felt when closed out of her relationship with her father. Although this was a defensive enactment, it was also an important one, as it enabled her to access the 'ruthless', 'evil eye' part object that led to a point where she was able to move from persecutory guilt to a more depressive position, where she could begin to see that her colleague's intentions were not purely malign, though without switching back to a paranoid-schizoid, idealised position where she re-cathected her aggression: perhaps she would never 'like' her colleague but could see that she was not wholly 'bad'.

As an infant, Ms. D. had been troubled by the vicissitudes of envy and guilt:

> It appears that one of the consequences of excessive envy is an early onset of guilt. If premature guilt is experienced by an ego not yet capable of bearing it, guilt is felt as persecution and the object that rouses guilt is turned into a persecutor. The infant then cannot work through either depressive or persecutory anxiety because they become confused with each other.
>
> (Klein, 1997, p. 194)

The recurring dream of the crow tapping at the window represented Ms. D.'s primitive fear of annihilation and replacement and her envy of the phantasised part object which had privileged access to her mother's and father's love and affection and played out in the transference as a precious object I was denied access to. Ms. D.'s intolerance of her envy resulted in the persecutory superego which split her objects as a means of defence. It was therefore important that her therapist and tarot reader were kept apart, along with reality and phantasy.[6] Although she knew it wasn't '*really*' true that her colleague had cursed her, she also *desired it to be so* as this re-created the original position of helplessness where she could be saved by a more powerful other, such as by the ideal boss who valued her so greatly before her colleague spoiled it all. Despite my anxieties that I was colluding with the bad object by avoiding it, my interpretation regarding her need to split her objects helped to contain her anxieties driven by the punitive superego and enabled her to confront it later in the session. A more confrontational transference interpretation would have quite possibly resulted in a borderline psychotic transference where I *became* the punitive superego.

In the countertransference, I somatically and emotionally experienced the isolation of being 'left out in the cold'. My feeling that it was not appropriate to turn the heater on – even for my own basic comfort – indicated a countertransference 'buy in' to the image of limited good, which dictated that at least one of us had to sacrifice something we actually needed, just to access the idealised object: warmth and comfort here only represented *commodities* that could not be shared in the brutally rigid zero-sum system of Ms. D.'s inner world. In a capitalist system, emotions are easily commodified and used, rather than mutually experienced and sensitively thought about. This was particularly pertinent to Ms. D., who had experienced both material and emotional poverty in her family. As an adult, she had become susceptible to symbolically giving parts of herself away as a commodity in an attempt to heal presymbolic deficits through a phantasised symbiotic re-union, perhaps here tragically signified by the 'advertising'-style terminology that she used as part of a protective false self (Winnicott, 1982). I think it was important, therefore – particularly given the power relations in the transference – that despite being initially tempted to do so, that I did not succumb to the seduction of asking *what the project was*, as this would have confirmed her phantasy of the transferential (mother) bad object – *a coveting, narcissistic evil eye that needed to know only for her own gratification*. This gave Ms. D. the opportunity to project *the needy* (child), *dependent evil eye of the one that needs to know* into me. It was then I who became helplessly left out in the cold, to 'have a dose of' what Ms. D. had felt in her own family and in unconscious phantasy. By refusing to tell me what the project was, although this was an act of defiant hostility, Ms. D. was able to draw an important boundary between herself and her objects and to communicate the difference between them. By making her therapist into the helpless and dependent infant, she thereby reversed the power relations to establish a more 'autonomous identity' (Benjamin, 1980, p. 148). This important reversal meant that Ms. D. was able to move from what Winnicott calls 'objecting relating' to 'object use'.

> This thing that there is in between relating and use is the subject's placing of the object outside the area of the subject's omnipotent control, that is, the subject's perception of the object as an external phenomenon, not as a projective entity, in fact recognition of it as an entity in its own right.
>
> (Winnicott, 1969, p. 713)

Ms. D. was therefore now able to 'use' the projective identification to render her therapist powerless in the transference, from *the one who needs to know* (for narcissistic ends) into *the one who needs to know* due to a sense of powerlessness (object relation in Winnicottian terms[7]). It was only when Ms. D. was able to experience the cathartic satisfaction of wielding this power in the transference that she was empowered to enjoy looking at me through the 'evil eye' and reverse the curse through experiencing her desire that I be given a 'dose' of her medicine. By expressing this rage in the 'facilitating environment' of the transference, she could then also reach out to her lost, benign objects such as the father who understood her. She could then introject and think about my interpretations and thereby access more ambivalent feelings towards her therapist and her objects (Winnicott, 1969). She could then begin to become more at ease with her 'ruthless' desire to compete with others and address her rage towards those who had benefitted from systemic inequalities (such as her boss), rather than those with whom she could potentially find more solidarity (such as her colleague). By reliving these early object relations in the transference and at work, psychotherapy had not only begun to help her to diminish the threat of the evil eye/ primitive superego but also to forge a new relationship with her objects consciously and unconsciously, in experiences of presence and absence.

Concluding Comments

In this chapter, we have seen how the metaphor of 'the evil eye' and the concept of 'the image of limited good' elucidate inequalities from socio-economic, psychological, and emotional perspectives which can deepen and enrich our clinical work. The case studies of the *buda* and Azande communities, combined with the historical research of Emma Wilby and the psychoanalytic perspectives of Jessica Benjamin, shine an important light on the shortcomings of a post-Enlightenment worldview which, despite its clear advantages, has tended to overvalue rationalism and devalue more intuitive and spiritually based ontologies. This defensive position has fostered the subjugation of such ontologies by continuing to mould them within its own image as a means of maintaining its privileged aggression.

This wider field of research has provided new and enriching perspectives which underscore the complexity of clinical work and the sensitivity it requires from the psychotherapist. As the case illustration demonstrates, clients who have experienced relational trauma and operate from the defence of the curse position may well also identify with esoteric or spiritual experiences that they wish to speak about freely. This may create jarring countertransference responses in therapists who may be tempted to easily write these off as defensive unconscious phantasy, which is likely to create unhelpful therapeutic reactions. Therapists therefore need to find means of integrating magical consciousness into psychotherapeutic work as opposed to defending against it through 'reality testing', which then becomes more about the desire of the therapist and also potentially colludes with an already hostile superego in the client. Psychotherapy therefore potentially offers clients a container and a live current where they may not only express hostility and aggression but, unconsciously and at a somatic level, know that one's subjective, spiritual, and intuitive experiences are as welcome in the consulting room as the material and rational.

Notes

1 For a full explanation of this myth, see Reminick (1974).
2 'Eating' appears to represent cause of injury, misfortune, or death rather than actual cannibalism.
3 The anthropological accounts I have read lack interviews with the *buda* themselves and the way in which they feel about their traditions and also their relationship to the Amhara and the supernatural.
4 This seems to allude to the 'sin' of giving birth to an illegitimate child and is therefore equated with witchcraft.
5 For a much more in-depth exploration of these ideas and 'dark shamanism', see Wilby (2013).
6 I do not suggest that one represents the other here.
7 It is important to note that Winnicott's use of the terms 'object use' and 'relating' can be confusing, as generally in psychoanalytic literature the meaning would be reversed. For Winnicott, however, 'relating' refers to the predominance of projection, and 'usage' means separation involving the capacity to see the caregiver/therapist as a separate person in their own right.

References

Ataria, Y. (2015). Trauma from an enactive perspective: The collapse of the knowing-how structure. *Adaptive Behavior,* 23(3): 143–154.
Baynes-Rock, M. (2015). Ethiopian Buda as Hyenas: Where the social is more than human. *Folklore*, 126(3): 266–282.

Benjamin, J. (1980). The bonds of love: Rational violence and erotic domination. *Feminist Studies*, 6(1): 144–174.

Bever, E. (2008). *The Realities of Witchcraft in Popular Magic in Early Modern Europe: Culture Cognition and Everyday Life*. Basingstoke and New York: Palgrave Macmillan.

Bourdieu, P. (1977). *Outline of a Theory of Practice*. Cambridge: Cambridge University Press.

Callow, J. (2018). *Embracing the Darkness*. London and New York: I.B Tauris & Co. Ltd.

Evans-Pritchard, E. E. (1976). *Witchcraft oracles and magic among the Azande: abridged with an introduction*. Oxford: Clarendon Press.

Finneran, N. (2003). Ethiopian evil eye belief and the magical symbolism of iron working. *Folklore*, 114(3): 427–432.

Fisher, M. (2009). *Capitalist Realism: Is There No Alternative?* Winchester: Zero Books.

Fisher, M. (2016). *The Weird and the Eerie*. London: Repeater Books.

Foster, G. (1965). Peasant society and the image of limited good. *American Anthropologist*, 67(2): 293–315.

Galt, A. H. (1982). The evil eye as synthetic image and its meanings on the Island of Pantelleria, Italy. *American Ethnologist*, 9(4): 664–681.

Hardy, T. (1976). The Withered Arm. In *Wessex Tales*. London: Macmillan.

Hutton, R. (2017). *The Witch*. New Haven: Yale University Press.

Klein, M. (1997). *Envy and Gratitude and Other Works 1946–1963* (3rd edn). London: Vintage.

Lacan, J. (2006). *Ecrits: The First Complete Edition in English*. New York: W.W. Norton & Co.

Lacan, J. and Miller, J. A. (2008). *The Ethics of Psychoanalysis 1959–1960: The Seminar of Jacques Lacan Book VII*. London: Routledge.

Lykiardopoulos, A. (1981). The evil eye: Towards an exhaustive study. *Folklore*, 92(2): 221–230.

Reminick, R. A. (1974). The evil eye belief among the Amhara of Ethiopia. *Ethnology*, 13(3): 279–291.

Sheldrake, R. (2005). The sense of being stared at part 1: Is it real or illusory? *Journal of Consciousness Studies*, 12(6): 10–31.

Van der Kolk, B. A. (2015). *The Body Keeps the Score: Brain, Mind, and Body in the Healing of Trauma*. New York: Penguin Books.

Wilby, E. (2013). *The Visions of Isobel Gowdie. Magic, Witchcraft and Dark Shamanism in Seventeenth-Century Scotland*. Eastbourne: Sussex Academic Press.

Williams, G. P. (1997). *Internal landscapes and Foreign Bodies: Eating Disorders and Other Pathologies*. London: Taylor & Frances; Routledge.

Winnicott, D. W. (1982). *Playing and Reality*. London: Routledge.

Winnicott, D. W. (1969). The use of an object. *International Journal of Psycho-Analysis*, 50: 711–716.

Chapter 10

An Alien Seed

Fear and Desire in Psychotherapy

Introduction

Building on the previous chapter and its elucidation of mismatches in power relations and its impact on clients, I now show how unconscious processes such as projective identification and the denial of magical consciousness by therapists can also exacerbate feelings of powerlessness that are inherent to the curse position. I reference paradigms from both psychoanalysis and the occult, with particular regard to Melanie Klein's 'projective identification' and Dion Fortune's 'psychic attack'. I have chosen these particular writers as – despite their apparent epistemological differences – each offers innovative perspectives on the aetiology of unconscious attack and its effects on the subject. Psychotherapy has hitherto tended to draw an arbitrary and defensive boundary between itself and esoteric theories of unconscious communication, but as this chapter and previous chapters have already illustrated, much of the clinical data we draw upon through 'projective identification', 'reverie', and 'countertransference' may also at times include forms of unconscious communication such as telepathy and other uncanny communications more typically associated with magical consciousness. I argue, therefore, that this border has now become essentially untenable, particularly as embracing clearly esoteric concepts such as projective identification whilst also making claims to its scientific legitimacy creates a 'professional hypocrisy' that Ferenczi astutely warned against (1994). This hypocrisy also sadly accords with an existing hubris of the mask of 'analytic neutrality', where projective identification may be attributed to the psychopathology of clients rather than their therapists. Each of these hypocritical aspects results in a potential scapegoating of clients who may share belief systems which differ from the therapist's. It is no longer therefore possible for psychotherapists to hide behind what Mikita Brottman calls the 'clinical cloak' (2011). Through a clinical example which draws upon the work of Thomas Ogden, I highlight the way in which 'reverie' provides essential data to make sense of enactments and what Grotstein calls 'countertransference complexes' (Grotstein, 1994). The clinical example also describes a client's striking ability to 'read' his therapist's mind in such a way that may be considered telepathic.

DOI: 10.4324/9781003168027-11

Unconscious Communication: Projective Identification and Countertransference

Neurobiological research has helped therapists to gain a greater understanding of the possible mechanisms underlying so-called projective identification. The Process of Change Study Group posit a pre-symbolic, nonverbal 'implicit relational knowing', which is part of a procedural memory apparatus existing between the infant and caregiver from the first year of the relationship (Stern et al., 1998, p. 905). This proto language underpins verbal discourse throughout life and therefore influences object relations and affect regulation. In his paper on 'mirror neurons', Vittorio Gallese writes that projective identification, transference, and countertransference processes are 'instantiations of the implicit and prelinguistic mechanisms of the embodied simulation-driven mirroring mechanisms' (2009, p. 531). Schore's (2011) research highlights the role of implicit, primary processes and the therapist's use of intuition, which contribute to a 'restructuring of the unconscious itself' (Alvarez, 2006, p. 171, cited in Schore, 2011). The acknowledgement of these pre-narrative factors in understanding the mechanisms of projective identification and the application of 'non interpretative mechanisms' is also therefore pertinent to the treatment of the primary curse, which is a font of unconscious phantasy and projective and introjective processes generated by attachment trauma (Stern et al., 1998).

As I have previously emphasised, treatment of the curse position targets primary process experience to address the implicit foundations of personality structure. This allows clients to re-experience elements of original attachment trauma in the transference, and/or the therapist may use other means of evoking primary process experiences such as the use of artistic expression. The interaction of attachment trauma and right brain–dominated unconscious phantasy stemming from the primary curse may also account for the *unheimlich* elements therapists experience in projective identification and countertransference (Freud, 1919). In such circumstances, therapists often feel somatically impacted in ways which they may find disturbing and indigestible and find difficult to make sense of. We cannot interpret what we ourselves do not understand.

Given the uncanny nature of experiences of projective identification and countertransference, therapists may also therefore have experiences which appear to transgress space/time boundaries, such as precognitive dreams and telepathy. Despite its significant advances, neurobiology alone cannot explain such phenomena, as it relies on standardised methods of scientific replicability (de Peyer, 2016; Hewitt, 2020). Therapists have therefore been required to draw upon theories from quantum theory and physics (entanglement, synchronicity), telepathic research (Sheldrake's 'morphic resonance'), parapsychology, and esotericism[1] (de Peyer, 2016).

Further investigation of these fields of research is beyond the scope of this chapter, particularly as I wish to focus on the work of 20th century occultist Dion Fortune with specific regard to her 1930 text *Psychic Self Defence*. Fortune's work offers esoteric perspectives that are not often included in academic publications on psychotherapy and ways of thinking about unconscious communication and psychic aggression that can enrich and complement our existing knowledge.

Psychic Attack

Dion Fortune (née Violet Firth) became one of London's first lay analysts at the turn of the 20th century, when British psychoanalysis was in its infancy (Richardson, 2018). As Fortune's career moved from away from psychoanalysis and towards occultism, she continued to reverently allude to Freud in her texts and maintained that esotericism and psychoanalysis could offer one another important clinical insights (ibid.).

At the beginning of *Psychic Self Defence*, Fortune recounts the details of a 'psychic attack' (2018). Fortune alleges that the attack was perpetrated by her boss at the time, a warden at the school where she worked. Fortune states that the warden's hostility was an act of reprisal, as Fortune had assisted other members of staff whom she believed the warden had unjustly reprimanded. The warden then summoned Fortune to her office and, after aggressively scolding her, repeated the sentences, 'You are incompetent, and you know it. You have no self-confidence, and you have got to admit it', 'several hundred times' for several hours 'like the responses of a litany' (Fortune, 2018, p. 14). Fortune wonders why she could not have simply left the warden's office, yet reading her account today, it bears the hallmarks of the effects of the immobilising hypnosis of both mind and body so common to similar accounts of traumatising attacks, where the recipient is frozen to the spot by a parasympathetic survival response (Porges and Dana, 2018).

> Why I did not pursue the obvious remedy of taking refuge in flight, I do not know, but by the time one realises something abnormal is toward on these occasions, one is more or less glamoured, and just as the bird before the snake cannot use its wings, so one cannot move or turn away.
>
> (Fortune, 2018, p. 15)

The way in which Fortune uses 'glamour' in this context speaks to the hypnotic timelessness of traumatic experience that it would take her three years to recover from. Fortune writes that her subsequent initiation into an occult order was instrumental in her recovery (2018, p. 18). She believed her alleged attacker to have herself been adept in the occult and came to understand from the experience that such attacks – in esoteric terms – target one's 'etheric double'. The etheric double 'receives and distributes the vital force which emanates from the sun and is thus intimately connected with physical health' and therefore accounts for Fortune's significantly depleted vitality and inability to move (Powell, 2007, p. 2).

Fortune attributes the most pernicious forms of such psychic attacks to the 'Left-Hand Path', a form of 'black occultism' which she regards as highly unethical and dangerous, as it is ruthlessly focused on satisfying the libidinal and unscrupulous needs of the magician (1967, p. 118). She posits that the driving force of psychic attack is 'telepathic suggestion', which manipulates the 'sub-conscious mind' by gaining entry to the 'soul', which allows the attacker to manipulate endogenously:

Telepathic suggestion is therefore a conscious magical act of aggression or 'forcible imagination' that relies on the skill of the practitioner, but importantly requires the sympathetic acquiescence of the object in order for the attack to be successful, as in cases of 'voodoo death' and faith healing/killing (Cannon, 1942; Gregory, 1952). Perhaps due to Fortune's personal experience of psychic attack and its devastating effects, there is an implicit understanding in her work that for already traumatised individuals, there is a greater chance of susceptibility to magical suggestion, particularly as they have become reflexively attuned to the needs of others. For the traumatised 'clairvoyant' individual operating from the curse position, the porous nature of the barrier between self and other that results from previous trauma increases the likelihood of the sympathetic vulnerability to this hijacking of the self, mirroring what already takes place in the subject's inner world. In such cases traumatised dyads unconsciously find one another and are attuned to wound or be wounded; a phenomenon popularly known as 'trauma bonding' where each split off unwanted aspects of the self into the other. These hostile exchanges then become repetition compulsions where the subject may not consciously desire an attack, yet a traumatised, *glamoured* unconscious 'double' (internal object) *wishes* it into an act of traumatic *jouissance*. (Lacan, 1981).

The Taking Over from Within

Although Melanie Klein's work belongs to a materialist psychoanalytic tradition, there are nevertheless some interesting parallels with Fortune's. Each was influenced by Freud and drew upon his work to develop their own theories and followers. Both were also interested in unconscious processes with a particular emphasis on the more destructive and aggressive aspects of the personality. Each also emphasise *the interiority of projection*: of *projecting into rather than onto objects*. In each case, the aggression begins in the subject and then drives the sheer potency of the projection and then *embeds* it – magically for Fortune or in unconscious phantasy for Klein – into its target. In Fortune's case, the currency of this aggression is black magic, and in Klein's, the death instinct.

There are, of course, key differences between Fortune's and Klein's respective models of psychic attack/projective identification. Firstly, the aggressor in Fortune's model is usually an occultist who consciously manipulates the object of the attack. However, Fortune also mentions the way in which telepathic suggestion can happen on an unconscious level in more prosaic settings, such as in the case of 'the panic-stricken soul of a selfish friend', which suggests a process similar to projective identification (Fortune, 2018, p. 35). In Klein's model, the 'attack' unconsciously takes place exclusively in the mind of the subject, and projective identification therefore happens in a 'monadic' unconscious, based on the phantasy of the subject projecting into and identifying with the *image of the object* (Grotstein, 2005, p. 1058). In projective identification, then, there is an omnipotent phantasy of 'remote control' of the object mother (Grotstein, 1994, p. 580).

Psychic attack depends upon the 'sympathetic resonance' of the recipient of the attack, which, as we have seen, is not applicable to Klein's model of projective identification, where 'object relations' are restricted to the subject's inner world (Grotstein, 1994, p. 580). Yet, as psychoanalytic thinking evolved after Klein, in projective identification, the 'magical thinking' of the child is no longer restricted to the subject but is seen to have a sensory and cognitive impact on the mother.[2] Projective identification now not only becomes an indicator of psychopathology but a means of communication that can be drawn upon by the therapist to heal his clients (Grotstein, 1994, p. 580).

This process of transformation begins with Wilfred Bion's paradigmatic revision and the introduction of a now dyadic model, now consisting of a preverbal infant who projects what is intolerable into his mother, who then responds to the projection. The mother attunes

> to her infant's feelings so that she can receive them, withstand their impact, and then translate them into appropriate meaningful interventions for her infant's welfare.
>
> (Grotstein, 1994, p. 580)

In Bion's paradigm, the mother's containing 'reverie' (2019, p. 36) transforms intolerable primary process anxiety ('beta elements') into what can be digested ('alpha elements'), which then form the basis of 'dream thoughts' (2019, p. 6). Importantly for Bion, it is *beta elements* which are the source of acting out in projective identification and 'are not felt to be phenomena, but things in themselves' (ibid.). With the introduction of the mother's reverie and these 'things in themselves', although Bion does not suggest that these elements can actually travel from one mind to another, *there is nonetheless the immanent suggestion of a psychic power in the infant which has a powerful impact on the mother*.

An 'Alien Seed'?

The Bionian (re)volution of projective identification continued with the work of Thomas Ogden. His concept of the 'analytic third' acknowledges the existence of intersubjective unconscious communication, though he also emphasises its asymmetrical nature, given that the focus of analysis is on the patient's unconscious (Ogden, 1997, p. 109). 'Reverie' also becomes a central aspect of countertransference which Ogden describes as 'the analyst's resonance with the patient's unconscious experience in the present moment', echoing to some degree Fortune's notion of 'sympathetic resonance' (1997, p. 77). This reverie enables the analyst to 'dream' what the client cannot (Ogden, 2009, p. 8). Ogden's work has revolutionised the way we think about countertransference as therapists. His profound reverence for intuitive right brain mental processes is conducive to work with clients who find it difficult to symbolise. For Ogden, the countertransference of the analyst is therefore granted much more clinical attention than in Klein's model. Ogden, like Bion, emphasises the pressure which is exerted upon the analyst through pathological forms of projective identification which may impact on his capacity to think (Ogden, 2009, p. 98). There is thus a parallel with Fortune's notion of telepathic suggestion, as there is a pressure placed on the therapist as if by 'remote control' (Grotstein, 1994, p. 585): the therapist is briefly placed under a 'spell' by his client. Ogden, like Fortune, highlights the ingressive hijacking of the object:

> In a schematic way, one can think of projective identification as a process involving the following sequence: first, there is the fantasy of projecting a part of oneself into another person and of *that part taking over the person from within*; then there is pressure exerted via the interpersonal interaction such that the 'recipient' of the projection experiences pressure to think, feel, and behave in a manner congruent with the projection; finally, the projected feelings, after being 'psychologically processed' by the recipient, are reinternalized by the projector.
>
> (Ogden, 1979, p. 357; italics my own)

Once again, the mechanism which leads to the analyst experiencing this ingressive hijack is unclear. There is also a notable difference here in the way in which the analyst responds to an attacking projective identification compared to the victim of a psychic attack through telepathic suggestion. In the latter case, there must be a sympathetically vulnerable aspect in the victim consisting of fear or desire. This results in 'piercing' the aura[3] of the recipient from 'within':

> the aura is always pierced *from within* by the response of fear or desire going out towards the attacking entity.
>
> (Fortune, 2018, p. 35)

Fortune stresses then that a psychic attack cannot have any impact on the victim unless there are sympathetic desires or impulses which respond to the spell. As she puts it, the magician

> cannot plant an alien seed. He cannot graft a rose-shoot on a lilac bush, for it will merely wither and die.
>
> (Fortune, 2018, p. 33)

Fortune compares this process of sympathetic induction to electrical communication and acoustic resonance. This perspective is echoed in the work of fellow early 20th century occultists Besant and Leadbeater in their 1905 work *Thought Forms*:

> In cases in which good or evil thoughts are projected at individuals, those thoughts, if they are to directly fulfil their mission, must find, in the aura of the

object to whom they are sent, materials capable of responding sympathetically to their vibrations.

(Besant and Leadbeater, 2020, p. 38)

In Bion and Ogden's model of countertransference, the analyst's 'congruent' response is not the result of sympathetic resonance or vibrations but the pressure placed upon him through a mysterious process of interaction that is not determined. As the mechanism of transmission is not explained, I would argue that this remains a mystical and occult process. However, given the asymmetrical model which Ogden emphasises, it is understandable that a response to a projective identification would not be attributed to the *fear or desire* of the analyst, as this would also perhaps indicate a need to go back into analysis and point to a corresponding questioning of professional competence. Yet puzzlingly, by not acknowledging that 'congruence' may be a result of fear, desire, or indeed psychopathology in the therapist, this therefore suggests that the patient has after all placed an 'alien seed'. This is problematic, as the analyst then operates from a privileged position of psychic 'purity' yet is so 'attuned' to his client that he can 'dream' what she cannot. This may unconsciously reinforce the perspective in his clients that their thoughts are toxic and unwittingly set himself up as a punitive ego-ideal and compound the curse position. Of course, we cannot disclose our own fears or desires to our clients as a matter of course, yet we must at least acknowledge to ourselves that, when we are significantly disturbed by our countertransference, our own fears or desires may be involved. In this sense, Fortune's work therefore proves to be instructive.

The 'Clinical Cloak'

If we do not look closely enough at the defences we sometimes rather cosily rely upon as therapists, jargon terms such as 'projective identification' become ways to shore up our defences and blind spots. Brottmann refers to this as a 'clinical cloak' that shrouds projective identification in defensive mystery (Brottman, 2011, p. xii).

> In the last twenty years, the term has been taken up very widely, and is currently used to refer to an enormous range of experiences and situations, both within and without the psychoanalytic dyad, so that its original meaning has become increasingly dilute. Most often, I suggest, it is misunderstood as projection that takes the form of simple scapegoating, and is applied to the subject (the analysand) rather than the object (the analyst).
>
> (Brottman, 2011, p. 95)

There is a danger that despite his best intentions, with the disavowal of the therapist's bad objects, he may scapegoat his clients. The 'clinical cloak' in this way serves to protect the therapist from an unveiling of his *own* fears and desires in therapeutic enactments caused by projective identification. It is important to note that 'cloaking' projective identification in pseudo-clinical terminology helps to distance psychoanalysis from accusations of mysticism despite the diffuse and subjective nature of the term. Therefore, despite its 'clinically technical' connotations, projective identification remains a mysterious and *esoteric* term. In the following example, this jargon is used to explain an occult process of a client placing what we may consider to be an 'alien seed' into the analyst.

> we could call this phenomenon 'corporeal projective counteridentification'. In these bodily manifestations the analyst responds to an invasion by the patient, who is placing an aspect of his personal experiences in the analyst.
>
> (Baranger and Baranger, 2008)

This example appears to be based on assumptions which not only make it difficult to dissect the way in which this corporeal transmission *actually works* but also how it differs from telepathic communication. It also adheres to the cosy assumption that if a therapist experiences a somatic sensation, then this is interpreted as a 'manifestation' of the patient's phantasy (alien seed). As Brottman affirms, although the magical aspects of projective identification are protected by a veil of psychoanalytic jargon, no satisfactory explanation has ever been offered as to how the pressure on the analyst is actually exerted (2011, p. 104). The following example particularly illustrates Brottman's highlighting of the 'scapegoating aspect of the clinical cloak'. In this example, an analyst experiences violent phantasies of disembowelling his patient:

> He thought, appropriately, that since he hadn't the least desire to disembowel his patient, the fantasy he had had must be a countertransference response to the patient's unconscious phantasy, and he interpreted the wish to be attacked physically (without, of course, mentioning his own fantasy that had motivated the interpretation). Suddenly, the course of the session changed, and an intense masochistic transference situation appeared, in which the patient identified him with Jack the Ripper.
>
> (Baranger and Baranger, 2008, p. 89)

Baranger and Baranger confidently opine that the analyst's phantasy '*must* be a countertransference response to the patient's unconscious phantasy', foreclosing the idea that the phantasy could be the analyst's own. Yet how is this 'must' arrived at? Once again, there is no way to *prove* Baranger and Baranger's hypothesis –short of asking the patient there and then – and in this way, the idea that the patient *put his phantasy into his analyst* seems to be as fanciful as the mechanism which put it there. The only evidence cited in this case to demonstrate that the phantasy 'must be' the patient's seems to rely on the analyst's conscious apprehensions alone. Firstly, Baranger and Baranger state that the analyst does not, 'of course', have 'the slightest wish to' disembowel his patient –I do not doubt that *consciously* he does not, for this would indeed be troubling – yet the assumption that it 'must be' the patient only amounts only to hubristic conjecture. Secondly, the patient's identification with Jack the Ripper I presume to have been evidenced by his conscious declaration, yet is it not also possible that the patient was picking up on a violent aspect of his analyst's unconscious which could also have conceivably *not* been the patient's or have been co-created? Surely both of these additional possibilities should have been entertained rather than automatically attributing causation to the patient's psychopathology. This clinical standpoint sadly colludes with the 'rational violence' that Benjamin conceptualised and which was discussed in Chapter 9: when the analyst sequesters his own fears and desires behind a 'clinical cloak' and attributes the affects he experiences to his patient's projected phantasies alone, he denies her the 'mutual recognition' which the already traumatised patient has been hitherto occluded from (Benjamin, 1980). As Hewitt puts it,

> People who have sustained trauma in their early development are acutely sensitive to the micro-shifts in the feeling states and attentions of others that would be imperceptible to most people.
>
> (2020, p. 63)

Hewitt highlights the near 'clairvoyant' sensitivity of the subject which, as I have previously illustrated, is an outcome of the interaction between trauma and unconscious phantasy that create a particularly doomed alchemy in the subject's psyche (Ferenczi, 1988). The 'analytic stance' of denying gratification and emphasis on boundaries may, of course, be appropriate for clients who rely on symbiotic defences, yet the default assumption that phantasies are always those of patients denotes a blindness in the clinician which contributes to unwittingly confirming unconscious phantasies of persecution and is perceived by the patient as a retaliation. It may be therefore experienced by the client as further evidence for the existence and intractability of the curse.

> Such dangers lie in the fact that judgments about what is 'really true' about the analyst and what is distortion of that 'truth' are ordinarily left solely to the discretion of the analyst – hardly a disinterested party. We find that therapists often invoke the concept of distortion when the patient's feelings, whether denigrating or admiring, contradict self-perceptions and expectations that the therapist requires for his own well-being.
>
> (Stolorow and Lachmann, 1984–1985, p. 23)

Therapists' donning of the protective 'clinical cloak' therefore points to a troubling disavowal that is part of an anti-therapeutic 'professional hypocrisy' which serves to shield us from the parts of the patient we cannot bear (Ferenczi, 1994, p. 158).

> In reality, however, it may happen that we can only with difficulty tolerate certain external or internal features of the patient, or perhaps we feel unpleasantly disturbed in some professional or personal affair by the analytic session.
>
> (Ferenczi, 1994, p. 159)

To work in the best interests of our clients, we therefore need to maintain an 'audit' of our own fears and desires and be open to ontologies which may not match our own. Clients who are magically conscious and hold beliefs in supernatural phenomena would, of course, not therefore benefit from stock interpretations that indicate psychopathology or even psychosis. Nonetheless, this takes place far too often and is often communicated in an underhanded and insidious fashion.

The Countertransference Complex

The post-Bionian analyst James Grotstein's work shows an openness to experiences which may be considered of a mystical nature. His writing also goes some way to address the problematic aspects of the clinical cloak through his innovative perspectives on countertransference and projective identification. He highlights the analyst's vulnerability to fears and desires, or what he calls the 'countertransference complex'.

> These feelings range, as mentioned earlier, from introjective identifications (emanating primarily from the patient), projective counter-identifications (emotional responses which the therapist is projecting into his/her image of the patient), and a host of other feelings belonging to what I would propose to call the 'countertransference complex'. Ultimately, the therapist's own infantile neurosis develops into a countertransference neurosis in conjunction with the patient's infantile/transference neurosis.
>
> (Grotstein, 1994, p. 587)

Through the identification of the 'countertransference complex', Grotstein acknowledges the possibility of sympathetic resonance in the therapist which leads to inevitable enactments. As a result of infant research and the wide acknowledgement of intersubjective processes in psychotherapy, enactments have now become important clinical material to be worked with and through. As Farber puts it,

> Patient and therapist can bring out the worst or the best in each other, in enactments which can enhance or destroy the treatment.
>
> (2017, p. 726)

Therefore, the greater the openness and humility that the therapist can access means less reliance on the 'clinical cloak' (which, of course, we all may fall back on from time to time). The approach which Farber and Grostein advocate means that when enactments (inevitably) take place, the therapist is less likely to respond in a fashion which scapegoats the client. The therapist, after all, needs to be able to be *wrong* at times in order to avoid the hypocritical enactments Ferenczi highlights. When working with 'cursed' clients who believe they have made the wrong moves all their lives, a sincere humility towards one's own 'inner selves' is a crucial therapeutic factor. This does not, however, mean that therapists should collude with projected bad objects. By experiencing enactments and holding in mind that we are participants in a psychodrama provides us with the necessary foundations to work through our 'countertransference complexes', so that we can become much more robust containers of what is unbearable to clients (Grotstein, 1994, p. 587). Despite the asymmetry of the relationship, this enables a working through of the patient's material in a way in which the client can *have an experience of 'mutual recognition'* (Benjamin, 1980). In terms of the curse position, this kind of transferential redress is crucial, as mutuality serves as an antidote to authoritarian superego phantasies and idealisations that result from relational trauma.

> Psychotherapy requires a collaborative working relationship in which both partners act on the basis of their implicit confidence in the value and efficacy of persuasion rather than coercion, ideas rather force, mutual cooperation rather than authoritarian control. These are precisely the beliefs that have been shattered by the traumatic experience.
>
> (Herman, 1998, p. 145)

Clinical Illustration: The Boss and the Banter

Mr. L. was a man in his late 30s. He had been working in the banking sector for several years and said that he found it 'completely meaningless'. He had also experienced problems with heavy social drinking since the breakdown of his last long-term relationship. He told me that he was fed up with 'always going down the pub with the lads from the office and talking bullshit'. As a result of his 'commitment issues', he had been involved in a series of casual and fleeting relationships, which usually ended due to his recurring infidelity. Mr. L. attributed his alcohol bingeing and infidelity to his love of 'forbidden fruit' which he 'could not help'. Mr. L. was an only child, and his parents were both in their early 40s when he was born. His parents were both devoutly religious and had always said to him that he was their 'little miracle' and that they were 'blessed' to have him. Although his parents would never say anything critical about any of the decisions he had made, Mr. L. always felt that they were disappointed in the career route he had taken and would have preferred 'something more scholarly and meaningful' than banking. His parents had also made complimentary comments about his cousins' career choices, which he had taken as a slight on his chosen path in finance. Whenever Mr. L. approached his parents about this, they denied that this was the case and told him that they only wanted the best for him and respected whatever choices he had made in his life. Mr. L. said on more than one occasion during his sessions that his parents 'turned a blind eye' to the fact he wasn't happy, which made him feel that he couldn't be vulnerable with anyone and that he always needed to 'be positive about things'. Mr. L. said that he hoped that therapy might help him to find work that was more meaningful to him and sustain a relationship without sabotaging it.

Mr. L. had been in weekly psychotherapy at the time of this session. He came into the consulting room 10 minutes late and slumped into the depths of his chair. He nonchalantly told me with a half-smile of satisfaction that he was still 'very hungover' from the previous evening. He then apologised for his late arrival and assumed a more earnest facial expression as if to communicate that he knew there was serious work to be done. He began to speak about how difficult it had been at work that day with all the demands his boss had placed upon him. He told me he had been unable to think properly; had a 'splitting' headache; and, to top it off, his boss had called an urgent one-to-one meeting with him as a result of his concerns about Mr. L.'s declining capacity to work productively.

There was a brief silence where I felt at a loss as to whether to respond at this point but which was then suddenly broken when he asked me with a worried look in his eyes whether I was annoyed with him. This took me by surprise, as up until this point I'd had no (conscious) reason to think that I was angry with him. In my mind, I had merely expressed the odd nonverbal nod and 'Mmm-hmmm' to acknowledge that I had been listening to Mr. L. I couldn't see how this could have been interpreted as anger.

I asked Mr. L. why he thought that I was angry, and he replied that he wasn't sure why exactly but that my facial expression 'just seemed angry . . . angry yeah and . . . maybe also a bit disappointed'. I was suddenly overcome by a powerful feeling that I had been 'caught out' and was under attack somehow. Was it something in my facial expression or body language that betrayed something that I was not conscious of? Had Mr. L. *seen through* my 'clinical cloak'? This sense of being 'found out' felt uncannily familiar, yet I couldn't pinpoint how – an indicator of the curse position in the countertransference. I then felt a twinge of anxiety in my chest, as if there was something of the little boy in me who had been caught out. In the brief but pregnant silence, I then had a flash of a reverie of this feeling of being 'caught out' by my staunchly authoritarian teacher at primary school.

[The following is an account of the memory which this reverie 'flash' relates to, and the affective nature of the memory is condensed into it. As Ogden affirms, it is difficult to accurately 'report' on moments of reverie, the chronological order of which is not linear, as in the case of poetry and daydreaming (Ogden, 1997, p. 77)].

Mr. S. had been writing on the board when a member of the class threw a ball of paper at him. The class giggled in nervous ecstasy for a few delirious moments. However, this would only last until we all realised that he had now stopped writing. Ecstasy then dissolved into a dreadful, silent anticipation, though he stood eerily still. He remained facing the blackboard, a deathly spectre suspended in silent fury.

Mr. S. then suddenly turned round in a lightning flash, his thin, wizened, and cruel face growing increasingly flushed with rage. His eyes were now narrowed for attack, and we all knew that his pursed thin lips only heralded apoplexy. He then asked, in a rasping whisper: 'Which little devil was responsible for this?' Quite

predictably, no one was willing to own up, largely motivated by the knowledge that
Mr. S.'s punishments were reliably severe and often had a sadistic quality to them.
The dreadful silence continued. Mr. S. then suddenly focused his eyes on me and,
with almost a smile, rasped again, now with palpable satisfaction: 'Monk! Why is
your face so red? You must have a guilty conscience!' I felt incredibly exposed and
weighed down at that moment, overwhelmed by the intensity of the time-stopping
stares of my classmates. I didn't answer Mr. S. as I had now completely shut down
in terror. I had expected him to pursue his line of inquiry, but he then mercifully
moved on to address the whole class once again. This wasn't a reprieve but cer-
tainly an escape: I had been let off. I don't remember if we ever found out who the
'little devil' was.

This primary school reverie had initially seemed incongruous, particularly as it seemed to me that I hadn't thought about it for many years. Somehow, however, it had led me to understand that I indeed was angry with Mr. L. This was not only for being late today – as he had been late on several occasions recently – but also because it occurred to me that he had again been late in his invoice payment this month, neither of which I had yet explored with him. I therefore also felt angry with myself, as it occurred to me that I had been avoiding addressing issues with him that may have presented a conflict. This made me feel cowardly and that I had been doing Mr. L. a disservice as his therapist. Moreover, the fact that Mr. L. had asked if I was angry with him somehow annoyed me even more because I felt as if I was being 'caught out' again – as I had with Mr. S. – though I wasn't the one who had actually done anything 'wrong'. Nonetheless, it seemed that my guilty conscience was a driving force in the reverie and the session: it was becoming a game of 'doer and done to' (Benjamin, 2004).

I then decided to tell Mr. L. that I did feel angry with him due to his recent late arrival to the sessions and overdue bills. I was quite hesitant about saying this, particularly as I felt as this might be perceived by Mr. L. as unthinkingly throwing accusations around as liberally as Mr. S. had done to me all those years ago. I was, however, surprised to see that Mr. L.'s eyes lit up, and he looked immediately relieved, as if my candour had taken a great weight off him. He said with a warm smile that he was glad that I had brought this up with him, as he felt that people were rarely honest with him about how they actually felt, and he knew that it was 'out of order' that he hadn't yet paid me for this month.

Something about Mr. L.'s move towards reparation felt premature, and I felt an uneasy combination of relief and the sense that I had 'got away with' something. This mirrored that of my schoolboy reverie, as here I became aware of a residue of guilt. I decided at this point that it was important to explore with him what this un-comfortable combination of guilt and relief in the countertransference might have meant for him. I said to Mr. L. that I had been curious about why he had recently been late with the payments and for his sessions, which had not happened before. He told me that he had been finding the sessions 'meaningless and not really going anywhere' and that this had 'frustrated' him. He added that he had wanted me to confront him, but when I didn't, it confirmed his idea that he had that I didn't care about him: like his parents, I was always holding something back, just telling him everything was fine. He added that not paying me and arriving late had therefore been ways of testing out whether he was right.

I said to him that it seemed that he was also testing out whether I also had 'commitment issues'. Mr. L. then laughed and sardonically said with a pointed finger, 'I see what you did there! You're also talking about how I can never commit to women aren't you? Well, you know why . . . it's forbidden fruit innit – I want what I shouldn't have'. He then laughed and 'knowingly' winked at me. I felt a pang of embarrassment. It felt as though we had suddenly become two work colleagues, and Mr. L. was inviting me to join in with some office 'banter' that celebrated his sexual virility.

I said to him that it seemed that we had both felt forbidden in different ways from being honest with one another and thought we might benefit in some way or get some 'fruit' from that. Mr. L. frowned, perhaps in annoyance that I hadn't joined in the 'office banter'. He looked confused and perhaps a little affronted. He said that he didn't really understand what I meant. I said that I couldn't help thinking it might be related to the mixed feelings he had had about not paying on time and arriving late for sessions. He said that he still didn't understand what I was getting at, and I realised that this comment was too oblique in this context. I decided to change tack and asked him if he thought that maybe there was there a part of him that wanted to get away with not paying and another that wanted to be found out. 'Could these represent two different kinds of fruit?' I asked. There was a pause. 'Like apples and oranges?' he asked with a mischievous look. We both laughed. Mr. L.'s frown, however, quickly returned, as if he was preoccupied by a powerful, intrusive thought. 'Yeah, there's probably something in that. . . . I guess I basically think that when it comes down to it, people really don't give a shit about me. Either they ignore me or bollock me like my boss! So yeah, I do things like that to test it out I guess . . . which is pretty embarrassing actually when you think about it, innit?' He looked anxious, and a little lost. He went on: 'I still don't *really* know what the fruit is though, man. Do you?' I now felt put on the spot, embarrassed, and somewhat lost. I had been improvising, and it wasn't working out – I was doing him a *disservice* again – *this accursed fruit was dying on the vine*. Mr. L. looked at me expectantly, but I felt I had nothing meaningful to say. I continued to feel embarrassed – my thoughts about what the increasingly evasive 'fruit' might be rang hollow in my mind. Mr. L., meanwhile, had changed his posture and seemed distant. He crossed his legs and placed his chin on his clenched fist in a moment of contemplation that I was, for a moment, now only an observer in; I imagined him as an aesthete from a far-off decadent time. His posture was rigid, and his eyes were looking at the adjacent wall, full of bitter rage: 'Well, you know what? I am thinking the way I'm going about things is essentially pretty fruit-*less*, isn't it? [The aesthete is still manifest as he theatrically points down at the floor to stress the *less*.] And I want other people to care, but they just end up proving me right *every – single – time* that they don't *at all*'. [Again, he is rhythmically punctuating the stressed syllables with his index finger.] He continued: 'Maybe *that's* the fruit, when I get that confirmation'. He then added with some acerbic satisfaction, 'But it tastes *bitter*, dunnit?' He uncrossed his legs and rested his forearms on his knees, leaning towards me. After a few moments of silence, he said, 'I mean, I know it's your *job* to care, but how do I know you *really* do? I wonder whether you'd *really care* about me if I didn't pay you, if you're really bothered if I don't show up as you get paid anyway'.

I felt the twinge of temptation to tell him that I did care about him, but then thought that in doing so I'd be showing him that I was unable to tolerate this projective identification which had tempted me to respond by 'getting away with it' – by resorting to a concrete answer that I knew he would not have experienced as sincere. I therefore instead decided to ask him whether, if I told him that I cared, it would make a difference. He replied immediately with an emphatic – yet curiously empty of affect – 'No, of course it wouldn't'.

There were some moments of silence, tinged with a sense of foreboding expectation. I said to him, 'It seems to me you feel like I have let you down'. Mr. L. resumed his 'aesthete' posture, now with his hands clasped around his right knee, rocking slightly as if ready for battle. He looked at me determinedly. 'You know what? Yeah, you did let me down. Why didn't you pull me up on it earlier? That pissed me off. That's like what my parents do, just please me all the time. Don't you wanna get paid?' He laughed. This was more 'banter', and I felt small: there was some scornful, even contemptuous bite in this comment despite its superficial, friendly jocularity – we were back in the office, and he was putting me down, like the office bully might. I was also struck by the harshness of his need for me to 'pull him up', which reminded me of a boot camp general. I wanted to confront this projective identification directly in the transference, but I was concerned he would have experienced this as retaliatory. Instead, I wanted to show him my separate mind which perceived his attack as a mirror of his object relationships: 'It seems that you are quite frightened of change, but every time you want to have an honest conversation with yourself about that, there is an inner boss who forbids you from even thinking about it – he pulls you up on everything you do. So, it feels like you're running away from this boss at work, but you've got this inner fight going on too'.

Mr. L. thought for a moment and then, looking directly at me, said, 'You know what? My mum and dad are sound people, and I know they care. Just it's always about the church this and God that and all about being "good" and "holier than thou". And I've never actually felt that I am. I've always felt like I'm *bad*, you know. So that's why that boss is there in my brain, and that's why I hit the booze 'cos he's *so damned mean* sometimes'. He heaved a big sigh and again looked at me expectantly: 'What am I gonna do, eh?'

He paused for a few moments and added, 'You're right. I do need to have a word with myself, don't I?' He laughed and his eyes invited me to affectively meet him – I smiled back.

There was the sense of becoming colleagues again, though there was now an awkward but tender vulnerability between us. I imagined us having met by chance on the tube journey home from the office after a tiring day. After some anxious, tentative moments, we find a mutual resonance in conversation, of beginning to know one another, without the watchful eye of the boss or the need for banter.

Discussion

This clinical illustration illustrates various processes of projective identification between therapist and client. The first of these is an enactment where, by not initially exploring the enactment with Mr. L., I became complicit in an identification with a split bad object: by confronting him, I would become his punishing 'boss' superego who would 'pull him up' for his attack on the relationship rather than raising it as a matter for clinical discussion, or by continuing to ignore it, I colluded with the narcissistic defence of 'getting away with it'. Like him, I was never truly free of a 'guilty conscience', as described in the reverie. However, as is often the case with 'getting away with it', this only represents an omnipotent phantasy of a complete escape from the persecutory superego as opposed to thinking about his own anxieties about his lack of direction in his career, manic binge drinking, and inability to sustain a meaningful intimate relationship. The severity of Mr. L.'s persecutory superego was a combined result of his parents' acceptance of 'whatever was best for him', his introjection (through their devout faith) that he must be a 'good boy', and their comparison with his cousins' success. All of these elements contributed to a psychotic phantasy that his parents were withholding a severe judgement which was continually deferred yet which might manifest at any moment in a dreaded but unnameable punishment, such as that threatened by my old teacher.

Mr. L.'s means of defending against the persecutory superego were typically 'diabolical' transgressions such as drinking, infidelity, and not paying his bills, all of which rebelled against the intolerant judge which he had projected into me. I therefore became his parents who were withholding their persecutory thoughts of retaliation. There was a parallel with the reverie – I became Mr. S., and Mr. L. became the mystery child who had thrown the 'testing' paper missile. It is pertinent to note that, in the school memory and in the session, I felt guilty for something I had not done but wished to. The reverie revealed a repressed wish that it had been me who had thrown the paper missile at Mr. S., which is what manifested at the time of the rosy cheeks of my 'guilty conscience'. I also felt guilty that I had not spoken to Mr. L. earlier about his attacks on the therapy and wished I had done so earlier.

In a further parallel with the reverie, when Mr. L. asked whether I was angry with him, there was a 'schoolboy' vulnerability that he transmitted that allowed me to empathise and identify with his conflicted desire to be found out but also to 'get away with it', desiring a magical solution *of being found without being found out*. These tensions were illustrated by the metaphor of the fruit. This, of course, evokes the much-quoted dramatic dilemma of 'hide-and-seek' that Winnicott describes.

> Here is a picture of a child establishing a private self that is not communicating, and at the same time wanting to communicate and to be found. It is a

sophisticated game of hide-and-seek in which it is joy to be hidden but disaster not to be found.

(1990, p. 186)

To be found but not found out denotes the confusion between unconscious phantasy and what Winnicott would call 'the environment': in phantasy, everything must be done to avoid the cruel superego – hence the need for id gratifications which promise relief but, of course, never will provide it as they too represent a danger.

Gratification brings peace, but the infant perceives that to become gratified he endangers what he loves.

(Winnicott et al., 1984, p. 89)

In my primary school memory, environment and phantasy had become confused. I wasn't actually 'guilty' of throwing the paper missile, yet I may as well have been. In my omnipotent mind, the culprit and I had become con-fused, and I was as culpable as they, as my hatred of my teacher was potent, which my burning rosy cheeks betrayed. I wished to triumphantly 'get away with it' but also, perhaps, felt that I 'deserved' to be punished for my 'evil' thoughts towards him and then be altogether free of them. This in itself equates to a magical ideal and is suitably indicative of the harsh Protestant dualism that Mr. S. was a proponent of.

My reverie was an important clinical stimulus which enabled me to tell Mr. L. that I was indeed angry with him. Initially, it seemed to me that my affective disclosure could have been framed within the confines of the 'real relation-ship', yet I think this would be a misrepresentation of relational dynamics, mainly because I also needed to show Mr. L. – in the transference – that his acting out had an impact and that I now saw him, and I was also no longer hiding (Gelso and Kline, 2019). This disclosure provided some initial relief for Mr. L. (and myself) at being 'found out', particularly as Mr. L. was able to tell me about his feeling that the sessions were going nowhere, which had been created by the enactment. Mr. L. then, though, quickly resorted again to the narcissistic defence (banter) and, by my not colluding with this and through his frustration at the conversation about the meaning of fruit, Mr. L. was then able to access the rage that he felt towards his parents, boss, and me in the transfer-ence. This also led to a further projective identification where he responded from the narcissistic defence of contempt and scorn. As I showed him that he would not destroy me and I would not retaliate, Mr. L. was then able to access some 'capacity for concern', here representing a third position between guilt and narcissistic defence (Winnicott et al., 1984).

We can see from this illustration how potent guilt and its vicissitudes can be-come in transference enactments. When I now reflect back on this example session, I notice that unconsciously I felt 'forbidden' from speaking to Mr. L. about his acting out but also a guilty feeling that I was doing him a 'disservice' and therefore *getting away with* something. By not initially confronting Mr. L., I was confirming his phantasy that as long as I got paid, I was not bothered, as I did not really care about him. This 'getting away with it' led to a confirmation that his therapist didn't care about him and a resentment (the obverse of guilt) in me.

Searles suggests that the guilt in the therapist may relate to 'unconscious empathy with the patient's child self-representation, who felt guilty about driving a parental figure to the point of madness' (Gabbard, 1993, p. 10). This unconscious empathy may account – in part – for my 'delay' in confronting his acting out straightaway, as I was unconsciously empathising with his fear of retaliation from a 'forbidding' persecutory superego (such as that represented by Mr. S. in the reverie) which he had (phantasised) that he had projected into me (Grotstein, 2005, p. 1054). This unconscious empathy is an important part of projective identification to pay attention to, particularly because – as we have seen earlier in this chapter – so much information is exchanged implicitly. This unconscious empathy also relates to the earlier discussion around the mechanisms of projective identification and telepathic suggestion.

This case illustration demonstrates the asymmetry of the therapeutic relationship and the conflicts that arise from it – in this case, with specific reference to fees and punctuality. Despite this asymmetry, there was also a sympathetic resonance between client and therapist as a result of shared experiences of hostility and persecutory guilt. It is important to note that Mr. L. also demonstrated his unconscious empathy, as he was able to sense my guilt and resentment before I did. Such levels of empathy can be startling to witness and are what come to resemble those attributed to telepathic and clairvoyant abilities. Fortune's theories around fear and desire and the 'alien seed' are germane in this instance: to me, it felt as if Mr. L. unconsciously knew what the 'seed' was, and he was therefore picking up on my fear and desire to be 'found out', and this was a point of striking sympathetic resonance that may be considered to be telepathic. Certainly, some of this fear and desire were the result of Mr. L.'s projection, but they were also undoubtedly in part my own of wishing to be a 'good' therapist and not do him a 'disservice' by being the opposite. There therefore was certainly no 'alien seed' here.

Concluding Comments

This chapter has emphasised the need for flexibility and sensitivity in order to avoid re-traumatising clients and compounding the curse position. Despite the obvious differences in esotericism and more traditional Western approaches to psychotherapy, the boundaries between them are not always clear cut, and the former can offer the latter rich knowledge in terms of interpreting unconscious processes of communication. The 'clinical cloak' offers a false sense of security which potentially fosters omnipotence and is therefore antithetical to what is most helpful to our clients.

Notes

1 For an in-depth analysis of these fields of research, I would thoroughly recommend de Peyer's 2016 paper.
2 I use 'mother' to generally represent caregiver.
3 'The outer part of the cloud-like substance of his higher bodies, interpenetrating each other, and extending beyond the confines of his physical body, the smallest of all'. (See Besant and Leadbeater, 2020).

References

Alvarez, A. (2006). Some questions concerning states of fragmentation: Unintegration, under-integration, disintegration, and the nature of early integrations. *Journal of Child Psychotherapy*, 32: 158–180.

Baranger, M. and Baranger, W. (1969). The analytic situation as a dynamic field. *International Journal of Psychoanalysis*, 89(4): 795–826.

Benjamin, J. (1980). The bonds of love: Rational violence and erotic domination. *Feminist Studies*, 6(1): 144–174.

Benjamin, J. (2004). Beyond doer and done to: An intersubjective view of thirdness. *Psychoanalytic Quarterly*, 73: 5–46.

Besant, A. and Leadbeater, C. (2020). *Thought Forms*. New York: Sacred Bones.

Bion, W. R. (2019). *Learning from Experience* (Maresfield Library). London and New York: Routledge.

Brottman, M. (2011). *Phantoms of the Clinic: From thought-transference to Projective Identification*. London: Karnac Books.

Cannon, W. B. (1942). "Voodoo" death. *American Anthropologist*, 1942(44): 169–181 (*Am J Public Health*. 2002 Oct; 92(10): 1593–1596; discussion 1594–1595).

de Peyer, J. L. C. S. W. (2016). Uncanny communication and the porous mind. *Psychoanalytic Dialogues*, 26(2): 156–174.

Farber, S. (2017). Becoming a telepathic tuning fork: Anomalous experience and the relational mind. *Psychoanalytic Dialogues*, 27(6): 719–734.

Ferenczi, S. (1988). Confusion of tongues between adults and the child – The language of tenderness and of passion. *Contemporary Psychoanalysis*, 24: 196–206.

Ferenczi, S. (1994). *Psycho-Analysis and Education. Final Contributions to Psychoanalysis*. London: Karnac Books.

Fortune, D. (1967). *Sane Occultism*. Wellingborough: The Aquarian Press.

Fortune, D. (2018). *Psychic Self Defence*. Naples: Albatross.

Freud, S. (1919). The 'Uncanny'. In Freud, A., Strachey, A., Strachey, J, and Tyson A. (Eds.), *The Standard Edition of the Complete Psychological Works of Sigmund Freud, Volume XVII (1917–1919): An Infantile Neurosis and Other Works*. London: Hogarth Press and the Institute of Psychoanalysis, pp. 217–225.

Gabbard, G. O. (1993). An overview of countertransference with borderline patients. *The Journal of Psychotherapy Practice and Research*, 2(1): 7–18.

Gallese, V. (2009). Mirror neurons, embodied simulation, and the neural basis of social identification. *Psychoanalytic Dialogues*, 19(5): 519–536.

Gelso, C. J. and Kline, K. V. (2019). The sister concepts of the working alliance and the real relationship: On their development, rupture, and repair. *Research in Psychotherapy* (Milano), 22(2): 373.

Gregory, J. C. (1952). Magic, fascination, and suggestion. *Folklore*, 63(3): 143–151.

Grotstein, J. (1994). Projective identification and countertransference: A brief commentary on their relationship. *Contemporary Psychoanalysis*, 30(3): 578–592.

Grotstein, J. (2005). Projective transidentification an extension of the concept of projective identification. *International Journal of Psychoanalysis*, 86(4): 1051–1069.

Herman, J. L. (1998). Recovery from psychological trauma. *Psychiatry and Clinical Neurosciences*, 52: S98–S103.

Hewitt, M. A. (2020). *Legacies of the Occult: Psychoanalysis, Religion, and Unconscious Communication*. Sheffield: Equinox.

Lacan, J. (1981). *Book XI the Four Fundamentals of Psychoanalysis*. London: W.R. Norton.

Ogden, T. H. (1979). On projective identification. *International Journal of Psycho-Analysis*, 60: 357–373.

Ogden, T. H. (1997). *Reverie and Interpretation. Sensing Something Human*. London: Jason Aronson Inc.

Ogden, T. H. (2009). *Rediscovering Psychoanalysis: Thinking and Dreaming, Learning and Forgetting*. London and New York: Routledge.

Porges, S. W. and Dana, D. (2018). *Clinical Applications of the Polyvagal Theory: The Emergence of Polyvagal-Informed Therapies*. New York: WW Norton.

Powell, A. E. (2007). *The Etheric Double*. San Diego: The Book Tree.

Richardson, E. (2018). Stemming the Black Tide of Mud. In C. Ferguson and Radford (eds), *The Occult Imagination in Britain*. London and New York: Routledge, pp. 110–128.

Schore, A. N. (2011). The right brain implicit self lies at the core of psychoanalysis. *Psychoanalytic Dialogues: The International Journal of Relational Perspectives*, 21(1): 75–100.

Stern, D. N. et al. (1998). Non-interpretive mechanisms in psychoanalytic therapy. The 'something more' than interpretation. The process of change study group. *The International Journal of Psycho-Analysis*, 79(5): 903–921.

Stolorow, R. D. and Lachmann, F. M. (1984–1985). Transference: The future of an illusion. *The Annual of Psychoanalysis,* 12–13: 19–37. https://psycnet.apa.org/record/1987-11041-001

Winnicott, D. W. (1990). On Communication. In *The Maturational Processes and the Facilitating Environment: Studies in the Theory of Emotional Development*. London: Routledge.

Winnicott, D. W., Winnicott, C., Shepherd, R. and Davis, M. (1984). *Deprivation and Delinquency*. London: Tavistock Publications.

Index

Aaron (priest) 7
affect, isolation of 70
aggression: examples in "Withered Arm"
  128–129; expressing in therapy 141; fear
  and 5, 8, 10; internalisation of 72; latent
  (Mr. F.) 117; Ms. A. 105; Ms. D. 139;
  in the 'Other' 130, 133; psychic 145;
  rationalism as defence against 130–133
aggressive 'badness', attempts to expel 81
aggressive behavior 71
aggressive defence 112
aggressive feelings 46
aggressor: identification with 70, 76,
  78–79, 86–87, 90; mother 91; parent
  aggressor, transference from clinician to
  69; pathological identification with 113
Aickman, Robert: 'The Cicerones' 63–65
Aiwass 19–20
alienation 39, 56, 73, 97; from own
  subjectivity 131
alien invaders, fear of 18
alien mutuality, sense of 104
alien seed 143–161
alien self 72, 75–76, 90
'alien sorcerers', magic practiced by 7, 10
animal magnetism 18
Apollyon 44
Argenteum Astrum (Order of Silver Star) 14
astral travel 19, 127
atman, the 15
Atonement, Day of 7
Azande tribe of Tanzania 124, 132, 141
Azazel 7, 113

bad luck 1, 4, 31, 43, 134, 135
badness 40; conditional 97; curse position,
  two forms of 108; expelling 81;
  internalised 114; Klein on 126; libidinal

97, 113; moral 133; *see also* burden
  of badness
bad objects 2, 33, 62; attempts or threats
  to 'remove' (via therapy) 69; child's
  ego and pact with 97–98; 'clinical
  cloak' and 149; colluding with 139,
  153; in Fairbairn's paradigm 94–99;
  Kleinian dialectic of good objects and
  83–84; libidinal attachment to 115; Mr.
  F. and 118, 121; Ms. D. 136, 139, 140;
  pathological libidinal attachment to
  105; people pleasers/saviours and 101;
  in 'Sandman' 59; secondary repression
  of 100; 'sense of guilt' generated by
  115; 'taken' into the ego 78; therapist as
  threat to client's relationship with 106;
  therapists' phantasy to cure patients of 99
bad omen 86
Baranger, M. and Baranger, W. 150
Beebe, B. and Lachmann, F. 37, 109–110
being evil 108
being in the world 132
being observed, phantasies of 111
being stared at, uncanny feeling of 125
being watched, sense of 60
Benjamin, Jessica 124, 129–132, 141;
  on instrumentalism 130; on 'mutual
  recognition' 153; on 'rational violence'
  124, 151
Besant, Annie 19, 148–149
Bever, E. 5
Bion, Wilfred 12, 147–149; *see also* Grotstein
Blavatsky (Madame) 14, 19, 21, 27
blood 81
Bloom, H. 113–115
Briggs, Katharine 85
Briggs, Robin 38
Britton, Ronald 84

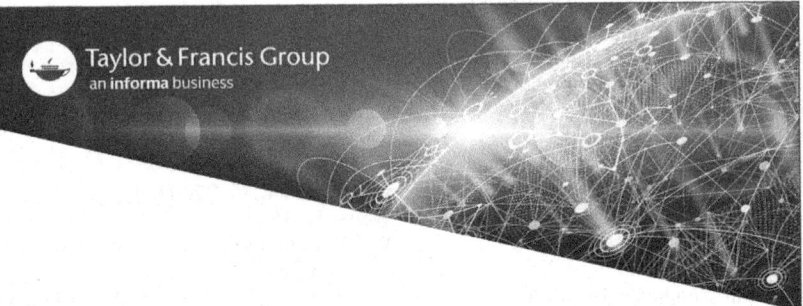
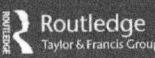
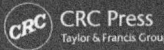